AF580872

MODELING AND DATA TREATMENT IN THE PHARMACEUTICAL SCIENCES

HOW TO ORDER THIS BOOK

BY PHONE: 800-233-9936 or 717-291-5609, 8AM–5PM Eastern Time

BY FAX: 717-295-4538

BY MAIL: Order Department
Technomic Publishing Company, Inc.
851 New Holland Avenue, Box 3535
Lancaster, PA 17604, U.S.A.

BY CREDIT CARD: American Express, VISA, MasterCard

BY WWW SITE: http://www.techpub.com

MODELING AND DATA TREATMENT IN THE PHARMACEUTICAL SCIENCES

J. T. Carstensen, M.Ch.E., Ph.D.

Professor Emeritus
The University of Wisconsin

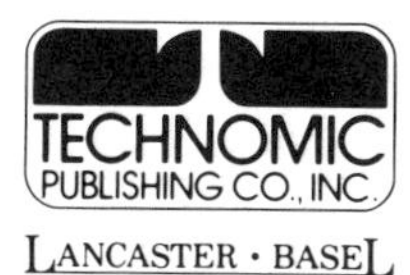

LANCASTER · BASEL

Modeling and Data Treatment in the Pharmaceutical Sciences
a **TECHNOMIC**® publication

Published in the Western Hemisphere by
Technomic Publishing Company, Inc.
851 New Holland Avenue, Box 3535
Lancaster, Pennsylvania 17604 U.S.A.

Distributed in the Rest of the World by
Technomic Publishing AG
Missionsstrasse 44
CH-4055 Basel, Switzerland

Printed in the United States of America
10 9 8 7 6 5 4 3 2 1

Main entry under title:
Modeling and Data Treatment in the Pharmaceutical Sciences

A Technomic Publishing Company book
Bibliography: p.
Includes index p. 265

Library of Congress Card No. 96-60624
ISBN No. 1-56676-440-8

With love, to my wife
Cathy Gene
(née Karr and still Karr), without whom the
book would have been finished much sooner.

Table of Contents

Introduction

THIS book has evolved over a span of twenty years, and started as a series of class notes in the graduate course Modeling and Data Treatment, offered biannually by the author at the School of Pharmacy, University of Wisconsin.

The intent of the text (and the course) is to (a) develop, with the student or reader, an ability to look at data and draw all the possible inferences from them; (b) evaluate such inferences statistically; and (c) then, most importantly, to form a picture, mathematically or not, of the actual process that is responsible for the responses. Hence, it has an aim to create an awareness of the use of statistics in pharmaceutical experimentation. This awareness transcends the rote use of canned programs in computers (and in the early 1970s contained no text on computers at all).

Aside from addressing the use of statistics and computers for data analysis, many of the examples in the book point to the *dangers* of such use without thoughtful understanding of the principles involved. However, the ultimate aim of the book is the ability to use data to *model* a situation, a phenomenon, or a process and to logically decide on further experimentation. The author has experienced countless situations where someone (a client, a student) would say that experiments were performed but that they were inconclusive, where, in reality, they were quite conclusive.

The procedures for modeling are outlined, and it is hoped that the reader who is *not* familiar or versed in modeling will become so through his/her visits with the appropriate chapters.

The book should be of use to anyone involved with preformulation, product development, process improvement, clinical data evaluation, and regulatory affairs, and it should be of great use to students and researchers in academia.

Finally, acknowledgements are in order, and it is primarily the research graduate students presently working with the author to whom he is grateful, viz., Mahdu Pudipeddi, Mandar Dali, Richard Schartman, and Miriam Franchini.

CHAPTER 1

Purpose of Pharmaceutical Research

THE purpose of research is to seek answers to questions, mostly by experimental means. Ordinarily, if one encounters a problem, the first step in answering it is to do a literature search.

1.1 LITERATURE SEARCHES

Nowadays, literature searches are mostly carried out by computer searching, and this is quite facile, except that it is often not all-encompassing. It is noted, for instance, that articles in the pharmaceutical literature prior to 1980 often had, to an abundance, literature references that were old, but few that were of recent vintage. These latter were accumulated by a conscientious following of the literature and, hence, depending on the time commitment of the researchers, would be proportional to the time s/he devoted to keeping up with literature. This had the disadvantage of not acknowledging more recent work at times.

In recent years, the trend has reversed since literature searches are good back to 1980 (because of the adequacy of key words) and only marginal prior to that. This has the disadvantage of some work being rediscovered, an example being the part of the work of Lu et al. (1994) (viz., the use of a cylinder to imitate the shape of a "real" crystal), already having been reported by Lai and Carstensen (1978) some fifteen years earlier, which is not to be found in the references of Lu's article.

It is always a good idea for a researcher to set up his own reference system, a method that, with special programs for personal computers, is fairly easy in this day and age.

1.2 RESEARCH MOTIVATION

As mentioned, research is usually initiated by a researcher or an organization asking a question for which no answer is to be found in the literature. In the case of organizational research, it is usually a commercial interest that sponsors the investigation; in academic research, it is (hopefully) intellectual curiosity (partly spun by a researcher "following the field") that motivates the undertaking. It must be admitted, however, that much academic research is undertaken for less lofty reasons ("publish or perish"), and there is, however idealistic one may be, always a bit of that aspect in research. Money is needed to sustain it, money must be sought, and in searching for finances, some influence on the field or direction of the research may sometimes be present.

1.3 NEGATIVE MODELING

There are several levels of modeling, and the following applies: sometimes a theory is reached because the opposite theory has been tried to exhaustion without success. Examples of this are

- the first law of thermodynamics
- the second law of thermodynamics
- the third law of thermodynamics

The first law of thermodynamics was a result of an enormous amount of effort to produce a perpetual mobile and the final realization that "it couldn't be done." This latter is usually a bad research attitude, but there comes a point, at times, where one cannot beat a dead horse any longer. The significance of such a realization, when it is justified, is enormous. It allows one to "get on" and draw rational conclusions, to develop a whole new brand of science.

The second law of thermodynamics is of a similar nature, realizing that one cannot make heat flow voluntarily from a lower potential (temperature) to a higher one in exchange for mechanical work.

The third law, that molecular motion stops at 0°K, is essentially deduced from the fact that temperatures lower than −273°C have never been accomplished.

1.4 HYPOTHETICAL MODELS

Hypothetical models are based on developing models from a set of hypotheses. Euclid's elements are of such a nature, the shortest distance between two points is a straight line or Einstein's relativity theory. They explain things in simple or complex form, but their proof is not possible, at least not at the time of formulation.

In a sense, this happens in the pharmaceutical sciences. Mukerjee, in 1965, postulated that the Corrin-Harkins equation would fail at high salt concentrations and that a salting out term was necessary. That this was the case was proven by Franchini and Carstensen (1996) and others (Mukerjee and Chan, 1993). This case is less so than the previously mentioned cases, because the point could have been proven at its inception, had it been followed up. (In fact, Mukerjee, through Chan, did follow it up, but many years later.)

1.5 STRICT MODELING

Modeling, in the strictest sense, is

(1) The visualization of the mechanism of a process
(2) The expression of this in mathematical terms (an equation)
(3) Showing that experimental data follow the equations developed

Much of the later chapters of this book will be devoted to this type of undertaking.

1.6 PSEUDOMODELING

Pseudomodeling applies to situations where one assigns a function to a phenomenon that is part of the visualization of the model in such a fashion that it will fit the data. The rationale for the function is not stated, but since the data "follow" the pseudomodel, one concludes that the model "could" explain the data. There is a bit of this aspect in strict modeling as well (e.g., the use of input functions).

Pseudomodeling also is the exercise of fitting experimental data to a series of equations from established models (Model A, Model B, etc.) and choosing Model Q, for example, because it affords the best fit of the data, and then saying that this is a diffusional process because it follows a model, Q, previously established for other systems, where the mathematical development was based on diffusion.

1.7 CURVE FITTING

Curve fitting simply implies that a set of data is fit to a curve (straight line, parabola, exponential, to mention a few), without an actual rationale for the selection of the function.

This type of exercise will be described in this book as well, and it is useful when

(1) Data are tabulated, e.g., instead of entering many sets of heat capacity data at various temperatures for many compounds in a table, the data have simply been fitted to a second-order polynomial and the table will give the coefficients for each compound listed[1]
(2) Computer programs are used, since equations can be one-line entries, whereas tables would require as many lines as data

1.8 ONE-POINT EXPERIMENTATION

This might seem trivial, but in pharmaceutics it is not. Products on the market are often the result of a "formula" that has been arrived at by empirical means; it represents a system in itself, and the problems with it are that of reproducibility.

The formulator found "something that worked," and although he used technical and scientific principles in his decision process, such a formula is usually not (although they may be) the result of the previously mentioned modeling approaches.

This type of system will be discussed further in later chapters.

1.9 REFERENCES

Corrin, M. L. and Harkins, W. D., (1947), *J.A.C.S.*, 69:683.

Franchini, M. and Carstensen, J. T., (1996), *J. Pharm, Sci.*, in press.

Lai, T. Y-F. and Carstensen, J. T., (1978), *Int. J. Pharmaceutics,* 1:33.

Lu, A., Frisella, M. E. and Johnson, K. C., (1993), *Pharm. Research,* 10:1308.

Mukerjee, P., (1965), *J. Phys. Chem.*, 69:4038.

Mukerjee, P. and Chan, C. C., (1993), *ACS Abstracts of Papers, Part 1, Coll.*, 206:164.

[1]This is, for instance, a practice in International Critical Tables.

CHAPTER 2

The Single Experiment

OFTEN, experiments are carried out once and no more. If an engineer needs the value for a heat capacity of a fluid at a given temperature (for the purpose of dimensioning a reaction vessel), he may simply carry out an experiment in the laboratory and determine the amount of heat needed to raise the temperature of the liquid by one degree. It can be done in a simple, crude calorimeter, and once it is determined, no more needs to be said.

2.1 DATA IN TABLES

Often, a series of single experiments are carried out, and in this case, material is arranged in tabular form. If our engineer, for instance, has determined the density for several solids, compounds A, B, C, D, E, and F, he might list them in tabular form, as shown in Table 2.1.

He might then use this, in a library sense, for whatever purposes the densities might be necessary. In other words, the data become sort of a page in a file, but this has the disadvantage that, fifteen years later, the file will be gone; hence, the work only served a purpose at approximately the calendar date at which it was generated. For data of this type, there is no publication medium (unless the whole project that sponsored the generation of the data was published).

2.2 CORRELATION

The more basic researcher might ask why the densities are as they are. The first step in such a situation is to seek trends, and this will be discussed later. Suffice it here to say that there must be some "molecular" reason, so it might be worthwhile expressing the data on a molar or a molecular basis. This is done in Table 2.2.

TABLE 2.1. Density of Several Solids.

Compound	Density g/cm^3
A	1.25
B	1.40
C	1.15
D	1.20
E	1.55

This is where plotting first shows an advantage. The data in Table 2.2 are plotted in Figure 2.1. It is noted that four of the points seem to "behave," but the fifth does not. This is the type of behavior that gives rise to scientific curiosity. The scientist may ask himself why and come to the conclusion that, in the fifth case, the molecules must be arranged less densely. He would then, probably, find out that A–D were of one crystal system with a given molecular volume per molecule, and E was of another system with different volume.

It is seen, therefore, that a type of correlation may be found, at times, when one-point experiments are carried out. It behooves the pharmaceutical researcher always to look for trends and to seek their explanation.

2.3 FORMULA CONSIDERATIONS

The most typical "single experiment" in Pharmacy R&D is the "formula." Pharmaceutical products on the market have all been "developed," which implies that there has been trial and error and that someone, usually the formulator, has arrived at a formula, found something lacking in it, changed it a bit, and so on until s/he has come upon the "best" formula.

In such a case, a series of formulae may result, and these are often presented in tables, and such tables are difficult to survey. There are a lot of ingredients, some present in one formula and some not in others, with

TABLE 2.2. Heat Capacity of Several Solids.

Compound	Density g/cm^3	Molecular Weight
A	1.25	313
B	1.40	350
C	1.15	404
D	1.20	420
E	1.55	388

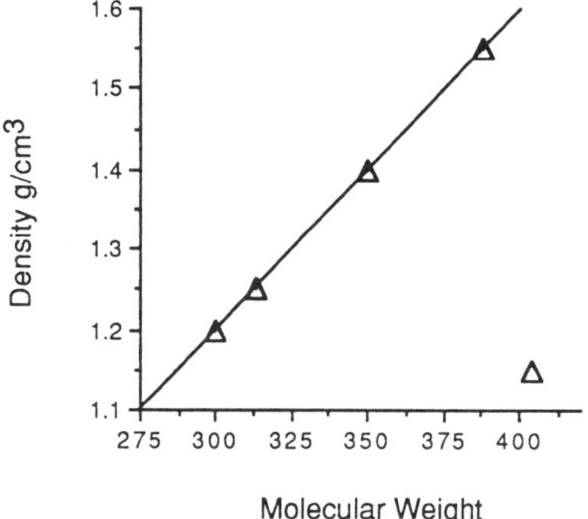

Figure 2.1 Plot of data from Table 2.2. The equation for the line through four of the points is given by $y = 0.003 + 0.004$ MW ($R^2 = 1.000$).[2]

varying processing parameters (compression pressure, amount of lubricant, drying temperature to mention a few), and to arrive at the "best" formula from such a set of experiments is difficult. An example of this is shown in Table 2.3.

It is noted that the formulator varied the amount of granulating paste which is being varied, keeping the overall composition the same. Tablets were then made from each of these and were compressed at 300 mg per tablet (containing $0.3 \times 6/1755 = 0.102$ g = 102 mg of drug per tablet). Usually, various attributes are measured, and various processing param-

TABLE 2.3. Four Possible Formulae for a Directly Compressed Product.

Formula Number	i	ii	iii
Drug	6 g	6 g	6 g
Corn Starch (dry)	170 g	180g	190 g
Lactose	1515 g	1515 g	1515
g			
Corn Starch (for paste)	55 g	45 g	35 g
Magnesium Stearate* 1/2%	(9 g)	(9 g)	(9 g)
Dry Weight per Batch	1755	1755	1755

*Prorated on Dry Yield.

[2]Least squares fits will be shown in captions in this book, with the coefficient of determination (the correlation coefficient squared, R^2) shown in parentheses.

TABLE 2.4. Hardness as a Function of Composition.

Amount Starch for Paste	Temperature (°C)	Hardness (kP)
55	80	18
55	50	12
55	30	10
45	80	12
45	50	8
45	30	8
35	80	10
35	50	8
35	30	8

eters introduced, e.g., temperature of wet paste, length of kneading, machine speed and a series of properties recorded (e.g., hardness, appearance, disintegration, dissolution). Results for hardness could be as shown in Table 2.4.

Several qualitative criteria can now be used. For instance, reproducibility is often the most important concern, so that if hardnesses of the above eight are satisfactory, then a content of either 35 or 45 g of starch in the paste gives reproducible results at all temperatures, so that less variation may be expected in such a case.

It is seen here that the judgment criterion is pseudoqualitative. There are, of course, other criteria (e.g., cost, dissolution, etc.), so that judgment must depend on all the *important* qualities.

2.4 SPECIFICATIONS

It is obvious, from Table 2.4, that batch size and the quality of the incoming raw materials are of importance. It is therefore necessary to set as stringent specifications on raw materials as the supplier can live with. This will be dealt with under the chapter section on factorials.

CHAPTER 3

Representation of Numbers and Data

3.1 TABULAR PRESENTATIONS

IF an analyst has developed the assay methodology for a new drug and has assayed all the batches, at NDA time, by this method, he might be asked to tabulate his results. They may have the appearance shown in Table 3.1.

The reader of such a table will automatically ask: "Well, what is the assay number in general?" and the logical answer will be the mean of the data.

3.2 MEANS

The average or mean, x_{avg}, of a series of numbers, x_i, is given by

$$x_{avg} = \{\Sigma x_i\}/N \tag{3.1}$$

For instance, in Table 3.1, the mean would be

$$x_{avg} = \{100.1 + 99.5 + 100.4 + 99.2 + 100.6\}/5 = 499.8/5 = 99.96 \tag{3.2}$$

Means, of course, may be calculated by hand, as shown in Equation (3.2), or a calculator or computer may be used. In most present-day situations, the use of the computer is the method of preference.

In this book, use will be made of a program[3] called StatWorks™. If the above data are entered into this program, the screen will have the following appearance after the data are input. That is, a column will appear, labeled

[3]Sold by Cricket Graph, Newark, NJ.

TABLE 3.1. Assays of a Drug Product at NDA Stage.

Batch	Assay (%)
1	100.1
2	99.5
3	100.4
5	99.2
6	100.6

Column 1. The assays are entered. (There is a "number column" where consecutive numbers appear each time a value is inserted in column 1.) One then types in "Assay" in the heading of column 1. One then enters the column headed Statistics and scrolls down to "Descriptive." A menu appears and one clicks on "Assay" and starts the program, and results appear as shown in Table 3.2.

3.3 THE DISPERSION

Our analytical chemist may, therefore, get into the habit of reporting his data by simply reporting the mean, and in the previous case, he might be asked: "But, how 'good' is the number you are giving us? How many times did you run it?"

In reporting means, one should always state the number of determinations upon which the value is based. This, in itself, may be ambiguous because the five numbers in Table 3.1 may each be a duplicate; hence, the

TABLE 3.2. Output from the Data in Table 3.1 Entered into StatWorks™.

Data File:	Untitled Data		
Variable:	Assay(%)	Observations:	5
Minimum:	99.200000	Maximum:	100.600000
Range:	1.400000	Median:	100.100000
Mean:	99.960000	Standard Error:	0.265707
Variance:		0.353000	
Standard Deviation:		0.594138	
Coefficient of Variation:		0.594376	
Skewness:	-0.177599	Kurtosis:	-2.062614

question arises: "Is the number 5 or 10?" The duplicate statement should state that the assays were in duplicate and that $N = 5$ batches were tested. This still does not say anything about the "dispersion" or "how good" the average number is.

3.4 MEASURES OF DISPERSION

Standard deviation (sd), variance (s^2), standard error of the mean (sem), and coefficient of variation (CV) are the means by which one answers the question of "how good" the data are. The abbreviations stated are the ones used throughout this book. They are defined as follows:

$$s^2 = \{\Sigma(x_i - x_{avg})^2\}/(N - 1) \tag{3.3}$$

In the above example, this may be calculated by hand as shown in Table 3.3. If the sum of squares is divided by $(5 - 1)$, then the value of the variance is found:

$$s^2 = 1.412/4 = 0.353$$

i.e., the same number as shown in Table 3.2. This, in essence, is one of the steps used in the validation of a computer program.

This serves as a good point to introduce the notion of the mean being the "best" number. Whether it is (e.g., could the median be better?) is not the question here, simply that the concept of best is often based on the least sum of squares or simply on "least squares."

As seen in the following, any number, A, other than the mean, will give a larger "variance." If one forms the sum,

$$SS^2 = \{\Sigma(x_i - A)^2\}/(N - 1) \tag{3.4}$$

then this has the smallest value when A is chosen, such that

TABLE 3.3. Calculation of Variance from the Data in Table 3.1.

Batch	x_i	$99.96-x_i$	$(99.96-x_i)^2$
1	100.1	-0.14	0.0196
2	99.5	0.46	0.2116
3	100.4	-0.44	0.1936
5	99.2	0.76	0.5776
6	100.6	-0.64	0.4096
Sum			1.4120

$$\partial\{SS^2\}/\partial A = 0 \tag{3.5}$$

But the left-hand side equals

$$\{-2\Sigma(x_i - A)\}/(N - 1) = \{-2/(N - 1)\}\{\Sigma(x_i) - NA\} \tag{3.6}$$

which equals zero when

$$A = \{\Sigma(x_i)\}/N = x_{avg} \tag{3.7}$$

The following definitions now follow

$$SS = \text{the sum of squares} = (N - 1)s^2 \tag{3.8}$$

$$s = \text{the standard deviation} = \sqrt{s^2} \tag{3.9}$$

$$s/x_{avg} = CV = \text{the coefficient of variation} \tag{3.10}$$

$$s/\sqrt{N} = \text{sem} = \text{the standard error of the mean} \tag{3.11}$$

The other terms in Table 3.2 are self-evident, except for the last two (below the line), viz., skewness and kurtosis. They deal with the type of distribution of the data and will be discussed elsewhere.

3.5 DEGREES OF FREEDOM

s is referred to as the sample standard deviation and s^2 as the sample variance. The smaller they are, the more precise are the data. It may appear strange that the sum of squares of the deviations is divided by $(N - 1)$ and not by N.

One reason that may be given is the following. If an analyst did four determinations and reported a mean and a standard deviation to his superior, the superior might want to try out another analyst to see if a better "precision" could be obtained. If this other analyst did only one determination and if the divisor were really N, then he would get an apparent standard deviation of zero because a number is its own average, so that the (sum of the) deviations equal zero. However, if the divisor is $N - 1$, then the divisor would also be zero, and it would not be possible to calculate the sd.

$(N - 1)$, in the case of averages and in general, the number by which the sum of squares is divided in order to get the variance is called the degrees of freedom, which will be denoted df textually and ν when used in equations.

It is, in general, equal to the number of determinations minus the number of parameters *calculated,* in this case one, since the average has been calculated (and used in calculations). In the case of a straight line, to be discussed later, both a slope and an intercept are calculated, so that in the case of regression, df = $N - 2$; for a parabola it would equal df = $N - 3$ and so on.

3.6 SPECIAL CASES OF STANDARD DEVIATIONS

Given the numbers 1,1,2,2,2,4,4,4,4,5,5, one might obtain the variance and standard deviation in exactly the same fashion as above. It is more convenient to do this in the following fashion.

$$\Sigma(x^2) = (2 \times 1^2) + (3 \times 2^2) + (4 \times 4^2) + (2 \times 5^2) = 128 \quad (3.12)$$

$$[(\Sigma x)^2/N] = [(2 \times 1) + (3 \times 2) + (4 \times 4) + (2 \times 5)]^2/11$$

$$= 34^2/11 = 105.8 \quad (3.13)$$

$$s = [(128 - 105.8)/10] = [22.92/10]^{1/2} = 1.51 \quad (3.14)$$

In general,

$$SS = \Sigma[(nx^2)] - [\Sigma(nx)^2/\Sigma(n)] \quad (3.15)$$

where the total number is

$$N = \Sigma(nx) \quad (3.16)$$

3.7 POPULATIONS AND SAMPLES

In the foregoing, it has simply been stated that a series of numbers or assays were at hand, and the parameters in question were then calculated. But these numbers are usually from *samples.* If, for instance, a batch of a million tablets were made, then the only correct number for the mean content would be obtainable by assaying all the capsules (and assuming that there were no assay error). Only in cases of nondestructive assay (radioactive count, for instance) would it be possible to obtain the assay of each and every unit of the *population,* as the batch would be called. The population, hence, is the totality from which the sample is taken.

When the mean and variance are calculated from the sample, we assume that they are good *estimators*, $E()$, of the population mean, μ, and the population variance, s^2, and we write

$$x_{avg} = E\{\mu\} \tag{3.17}$$

and

$$s^2 = E\{\sigma^2\} \tag{3.18}$$

To illustrate this, the following, somewhat extreme example is used—extreme, because for computational purposes, it is only manageable to use a batch size that is small and a sampling scheme that results in only a limited amount of sample possibilities.

We will assume that we have made a batch of twelve capsules for a trial of only one person. We need one capsule for our clinical trial and want to be as sure as possible that we have a good value for the estimated content. Hence, we use the remaining eleven capsules for assay and assay them individually. We will assume that there is no analytical error.

Again, we do not know the content of all twelve capsules, only the eleven we have sampled. The actual population (twelve capsules) is shown in Table 3.4.

If the first capsule had been used for the trial, then the sample would have had the make-up shown in Column #3; if the second had been used,

TABLE 3.4. Actual Contents of a Batch of Twelve Capsules.

Capsule Number	Actual Content (% LC)	Sample #1	Sample #2
1	104.5		104.5
2	102.5	102.5	
3	102	102	102
4	101	101	101
5	100.7	100.7	100.7
6	100.1	100.1	100.1
7	99.9	99.9	99.9
8	99.3	99.3	99.3
9	99	99	99
10	98	98	98
11	97.5	97.5	97.5
12	95.5	95.5	95.5

LC will be used as an abbreviation for Label Claim throughout the book.

TABLE 3.5. Means and Standard Deviations of the Eleven Possible Samples from Table 3.4.

Sample	Mean	Standard Dev.
0*	100	2.412
1	99.59	2.047
2	99.77	2.391
3	99.82	2.442
4	99.91	2.508
5	99.94	2.519
6	99.99	2.530
7	100.01	2.530
8	100.06	2.519
9	100.09	2.508
10	100.23	2.391
11	100.41	2.047
Average	99.98	2.403
Variance	0.0495	0.03365
Standard Dev.	0.222	0.183

*Refers to population, not sample.

then the sample would have been as shown in Column #4, and samples of this type have been constructed for the eleven possibilities of sample of size (12 − 1) = 11 units.

The (sample) mean and (sample) standard deviation are listed for each of these in Table 3.5. The data in Table 3.5 are what is denoted as normally distributed (or nearly so). This type of data will be the subject of discussion at a later point.

It is seen that the samples are good estimates of the population average. The standard deviations are also good estimates of the population standard deviation (2.40 versus 2.41). It is noted that the standard deviation of the averages is considerably smaller than the sample standard deviation. The sample here is too small for quantitative conclusions, but this phenomenon (the *t*-distribution) will be the subject of a later chapter. It is also noted that the standard deviation itself has a standard deviation, i.e., is not an absolute number. This will also be a subject of a later chapter.

3.8 THE POOLED STANDARD DEVIATION

Often, the question arises that, if one has several sets of the same type of, say, assays, each with a certain standard deviation, what would be the best number for the "average" standard deviation?

It is a statistical convention to add variances and divide by the number of degrees of freedom. If, for instance, Set A had four values and a standard deviation of 1.5, Set B had five values and a standard deviation of 2, and Set C had three values and a standard deviation of 1.1, then the total number of degrees of freedom would be

$$df = (4 - 1) + (5 - 1) + (3 - 1) = 9 \tag{3.19}$$

and the weighted sum of the variances would be

$$\Sigma s^2 = 3 \cdot 2.25 + 4 \cdot 4 + 2 \cdot 1.21 = 6.75 + 16 + 2.42 = 25.17 \tag{3.20}$$

so that the "best" value for the standard deviation would be

$$s_{pooled} = \{25.17/9\}^{1/2} = \sqrt{2.8} = 1.58 \tag{3.21}$$

It is noted that it is between the extremes of 1.1 and 2 but that it is not the average of 2, 1.5, and 1.1 (average being 1.53).

3.8.1 EXAMPLE 3.1

Given the set of data in Table 3.6, calculate the pooled standard deviation.

3.8.2 ANSWER 3.1

The pooled standard deviation is given by

TABLE 3.6. Quality Control Assays from Four Batches.

	Assay A	Assay B	Assay C	Assay D	
	15.2	14.2	13.2	13.2	
	15.0	14.9	13.0	13.0	
	15.8	14.9	13.8	13.8	
	14.2	15.0	14.2	14.2	
		14.5		14.5	
		14.8		14.7	
s^2	0.436	0.094	0.303	0.480	
N-1	3	5	3	5	Σ= 16
SS	1.31	0.47	0.91	2.4	Σ =5.09

$$s^2_{\text{pooled}} = \Sigma SS_i / \Sigma(N_i - 1) \qquad (3.22)$$

where SS_i refers to the sums of squares from the *i*th columns and N_i refers to the number of data points in each column. In the case in Table 3.6, this would be

$$s^2_{\text{pooled}} = 5.09/16 = 0.318 \qquad (3.23)$$

$$s_{\text{pooled}} = [0.318]^{1/2} = 0.56 \qquad (3.24)$$

3.9 PROBLEM

(1) As a scientist, in what other scientific branch have you encountered the term *degrees of freedom?*

3.10 ANSWER

(1) Gibbs's phase rule. Here, however, df has another meaning.

CHAPTER 4

Computer Programs

IT is rare, nowadays, that calculations of any kind are made by hand. Calculators, of course, are used a lot, but for more complicated calculations, these, too, are time-consuming so that it is customary to program problems of even moderate complexity.

4.1 DATA GENERATION FROM EQUATIONS, BASIC

The program language that will be used in this book is BASIC. It is one of the oldest languages, but it is easy to handle (anyone can self-learn it), and for this reason it is applied. The most important functions are discussed briefly below.

4.1.1 INPUT

This function allows a chosen value to be inserted in the program. It may be followed by a comma, in which case, when the program is run, a "?" will appear. For clarity, particularly if there are many inputs, it is customary to number the lines (starting with 100) and make sequences of 10 and to follow the INPUT command with "Variable="; X1 where the variable is what is being input. Whenever X1 appears in the program, it refers to this variable. In that case, when the program is run,

VARIABLE=

will appear on the screen, and the value is then typed in.

200 **FOR** X1 = 0 **TO** Z, **STEP** Q

. . .

1000 **NEXT X1**

is a useful command that allows generation of data points if a function is known. The following is a necessary command when data are being generated for a **FOR/NEXT** command as shown above:

300 **PRINT** X1, Y1

It will, *on the screen,* show the *X,Y* values aimed at in the previous program. For print-out, a dot matrix printer can be activated to print out the data, but in this case the command has to be

300 LPRINT X1, Y1

Headings of tables may be placed after the INPUT commands by simply adding a command:

PRINT "X", "Y" or **LPRINT** "X", "Y"

It is noted that symbols and phrases placed in quotes will print out (what is between the quotation marks).

4.1.2 EXAMPLE 4.1

Write a program to generate *y*-values for the equation:

$$y = a + bx + cx^2 \tag{4.1}$$

in such a way that data can be generated for N values of x and for any desired value of a, b, and c.

TABLE 4.1. Program for Equation (4.1).

```
100 INPUT "A="; A
110 INPUT "B="; B
120 INPUT "C="; C
130 INPUT "NO OF STEPS="; N
140 INPUT "MIN X-VALUE="; X1
150 INPUT "MAX X-VALUE="; X2
160 Z1 = (X2-X1)/N
170 PRINT "X","Y"
200 FOR X3 = X1 TO X2 STEP Z1
210 Y = A + (B*X3) + (C*(X3^2))
220 PRINT X3,Y
300 NEXT X3
```

4.1.3 ANSWER 4.1

The appropriate program is shown in Table 4.1. Of course, any equation could be placed in Step 210.

When the program is run, the following output results on the screen:

Values Input On Computer:	
A=? 1	
B=? 1.5	
C = 2	
No Steps=? 10	
Min X-value=? 0	
Max X-value =? 10	
Print-Out On Screen After Command To Run:	
X	Y
0	1
1	4.5
2	12
3	23.5
4	39
5	58.5
6	82
7	109.5
8	141
9	176.5
10	216

The command LPRINT would have to be used in steps 170 and 220 for the results to print out on a printer (dot-matrix printer).

4.2 STATWORKS™

Although statistical programs can be written in BASIC, there are occasions, many in fact, where rapid statistical analysis is in order. For such purposes, the program used in this text is StatWorks™.

As an example, assume that, after the first five batches of a product has been produced, the assays in Table 4.2 were obtained. These data are en-

TABLE 4.2. Assays of Batches.

Batch #		2	3	4	5	6
Assay	100	101	99.5	100.2	99.2	101.2

TABLE 4.3. StatWorks™ Output of Data in Table 4.2.

```
Data File: Table 4.3
Variable: Initial Assay          Observations: 6
------------------------------------------------------------
Minimum: 99.200000               Maximum: 101.200000
Range:    2.000000               Median:  100.100000
------------------------------------------------------------
Mean: 100.183333     Standard Error: 0.324979
------------------------------------------------------------
Variance:                        0.633667
Standard Deviation:              0.796032
Coefficient of Variation:        0.794575
------------------------------------------------------------
Skewness:   0.105549             Kurtosis: -1.892863
```

tered in a column in StatWorks™ and under the heading *Stat,* the address *Descriptive* is highlighted and run. This results in the screen (or print) output shown in Table 4.3.

There are a series of options (regression, ordering in ascending or descending order, etc.) that will be referred to as the text proceeds.

The output from StatWorks™ may be imported into programs (by using the Grab option under Edit) such as Microsoft Word™ so that results can be printed directly within a text.

4.3 SIGMAPLOT® [4]

For a nonlinear fitting and regression, the program SigmaPlot® will be used occasionally. Again, for this program, the reader is referred to the manual. SigmaPlot® is user-friendly. It contains a series of transforms that offer the advantage that the actual program used for the operation can be brought out on a screen, so that the user may acquaint himself with whatever shortcuts are used. An example of this is the program that allows least squares fitting with confidence bounds. As shall be discussed later, it is often advantageous to approximate the student t-values by a continuous function, which can be easily handled programwise. The SigmaPlot® program reveals the use of a seventh-order polynomial for this.

[4]Norby, J., Rubenstein, S., Tuerke, T., Farmer, C. S., Forood, R. and Bennington, J., (1990): SigmaPlot® Scientific Graph System, MAC, Transforms and Curve Fitting. Jandel Scientific, Tel.: (415)453-6700.

4.4 GRAPHICAL PROGRAM (CRICKETGRAPH™)

For data presentation, CricketGraph™ is used throughout this text. CricketGraph™ is user-friendly and gives good graph and some parameter estimations (e.g., least squares fits).

CricketGraph™ graphics may be imported into documents such as Microsoft Word® [5] by using the copy command under Edit. Columns may be copied into texts, one by one, as well. The program offers options of fonts and sizes, and writing can be added to the graph, and the size of the graph can be changed to suit the intended purpose. Legends can be left in or out as desired.

[5]Microsoft Word is a registered trademark of Microsoft, Inc.

CHAPTER 5

Curve Fitting and Phenomenology

TABULATING and merely plotting data on graph paper are the first steps in a logical presentation of results from experimentation, compilation, and a literature search. But for data to be of value, it must be possible to draw conclusions from them. In the simplest case, one might want to extrapolate data to some given value, and this is best accomplished by *curve fitting*. An example of this would be if one had drawn a curve of the amount of drug remaining in a dosage form as a function of storage time and had plotted data up to 12 months. One might then ask: How much would remain after 24 months? One could assume linearity and predict that twice as much would degrade in two years, but the question would arise if it would be wise to assume linearity. One therefore attempts to find a best equation, a curve, that fits the data best.

This curve may have nothing at all to do with what the theoretical curve should be, but it allows the practical task of extrapolation in its simplest form.

The next logical step is to ask whether the curve is logical. One might, for instance, find that the decomposition equation is zero-order, i.e., that the amount remaining after time t is

$$C = C_0 - kt \tag{5.1}$$

but it is obvious that this equation cannot be universally true, because when $t > C_0/k$, the "concentration" would be negative. This will be discussed later.

In the case of particle size distributions, it has often been stated that they should be log-probability. The point is that this has been found empirically, but one may have made the assumption that the particles have sizes from zero to infinity, i.e., that there is an infinitely small probability of having a boulder in the sample. Imposing rational limits on the distribution is part of phenomenology.

The point is that, if the scientist starts questioning the form of the curve and selecting one curve over and above another one (which may afford a statistically better fit), then he enters the realm of phenomenology. Phenomenology, hence, is the fitting of data to an equation selected with a view towards initial and boundary conditions or selected with some physical restraint in mind.

5.1 CURVE FITTING OF CONTINUOUS CURVES

In cases where one wants to present a continuous curve (e.g., a spectral curve, optical density versus wavelength), the experimental data a scientist obtains constitute a continuous curve. This represents an infinite number of points, and it should be pointed out that such curves can be (almost) exactingly represented by Fourier series, i.e.,

$$y = a_o + \Sigma a_i \cos [it] + \Sigma b_i \sin [it] \tag{5.2}$$

There are other presentation modes that fit such curves, but the problem that will be addressed in this text is that of fitting curves to experimental data where a limited amount of data points are available.

5.2 CURVE FITTING

Aside from the (mathematically) simplest of cases, which is to make a system reproducible and giving a recipe for so doing, the next step that occurs in data gathering is curve fitting. It is assumed below that a set of variables have been found to be significant, e.g., by factorial experimentation.

5.3 CURVE FITTING BY COMPUTER GRAPHING PROGRAMS

CricketGraph™ is the graphics data program used in this text. It allows fitting of data to curves as shall be shown in the following. A set of solid-state stability data for one batch is given in Table 5.1.

If these data are entered into CricketGraph™ (version 2.0), then a command in Scatter Plot will produce the trace in Figure 5.1. It is seen (in the legend) that the fit is good. (At this point, it should simply be mentioned that, when R^2 is close to one, the fit is good. The meaning of this statement and its limitation will be dealt with later.)

TABLE 5.1. Data for the Decomposition of a Drug in a Solid Dosage Form.

Time (Years)	Percent of Label Claim
0	100.1
0.5	98.6
1.0	98.1
1.5	97.1
2.0	95.5
2.5	95
3.0	94

The equation for the line given by the program is

$$\% \text{ Retained} = 99.925 - 2.0071x \tag{5.3}$$

This, of course, allows the user to obtain a calculated % LC at any time, e.g., if it were desired to know what the strength would be after 4 years, one simply inserts $x = 4$ and obtains

$$\% \text{ Retained} = 99.925 - 8.0284 = 91.9\% \text{ LC} \tag{5.4}$$

But extrapolations are, first of all, dangerous. How does one really know that the data will follow a straight line beyond the last point? Even if one

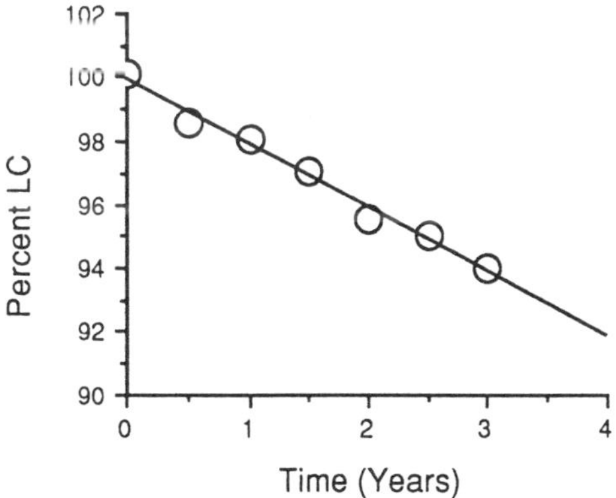

Figure 5.1 Data from Table 5.1 plotted zero-order. The least squares fit is $y = 99.925 - 2.0071x$ ($R^2 = 0.986$).

assumes linearity, there is a flaw in the presentation. If one asked what the potency would be after 50 years, one would obtain the answer:

$$99.925 - 100.355 = -0.43\% \text{ LC} \tag{5.5}$$

This, of course, is ridiculous, and the answer is that, after 99.925/2.0071 = 49.8 years, the potency will be zero so the correct equation is

$$y = 99.925 - 2.0071x \qquad 0 < x < 49.8 \tag{5.6}$$

$$y = 0 \qquad x > 49.8 \tag{5.7}$$

5.4 DOMAINS

This points out the importance of defining the domain in which an equation applies. Usually it is not of importance, but at times it is, and it is good practice always to include it in one's reporting.

There are many other examples where it is even more germane; e.g., in dissolution, the polydisperse dissolution equation can only hold until the smallest particle has dissolved.

5.5 SELECTION OF ORDINATE AND ABSCISSA

The example in Figure 5.1 was from one particular batch of tablets. Often, many sets of data are present, and it is important to show whether the data are linear or curved. For this reason and also for being able to show many data findings in one graph, it is important to be able to consolidate one's results.

Take the results from Table 5.1, but with two or more batches included. These data are shown in Table 5.2.

A lot of assay work has, obviously, been done, and it would be desirable to show all these figures in one graph. If this is simply done by entering the data into CricketGraph™, then a graph such as shown in Figure 5.2 results.

To normalize all these data, it is first necessary to unify the y-axis. This is done by expressing all the data in fraction retained.[6] This is done easily in CricketGraph™, since under the address *Data,* the subaddress *Simple*

[6]It should be noted that the FDA stability guidelines do not permit this. This treatment is strictly investigational.

TABLE 5.2. Data for the Decomposition of a Drug in a Solid Dosage Form.

Time (Years)	Percent of Label Claim			
	Batch A	Batch B	Batch C	Batch D
0	100.1	101	99	102
0.5	98.6	97	97	100
1.0	98.1	94.2	95.6	100
1.5	97.1	89	93	99
2.0	95.5	84	91	97
2.5	95			95
3.0	94			

Math, allows the division immediately for the entire column. When this is carried out, the data in Table 5.3 result.

If the data are presented by fraction retained,[7] then the figures in Table 5.3 result and the graph becomes as shown in Figure 5.3.

One may now calculate the time,[8] t_{90}, it takes for the strength to fall to 90%, i.e., a fraction of 0.9. For example, for Batch A,

$$0.9 = 0.99825 - 2.0051 \cdot t_{90} \tag{5.8}$$

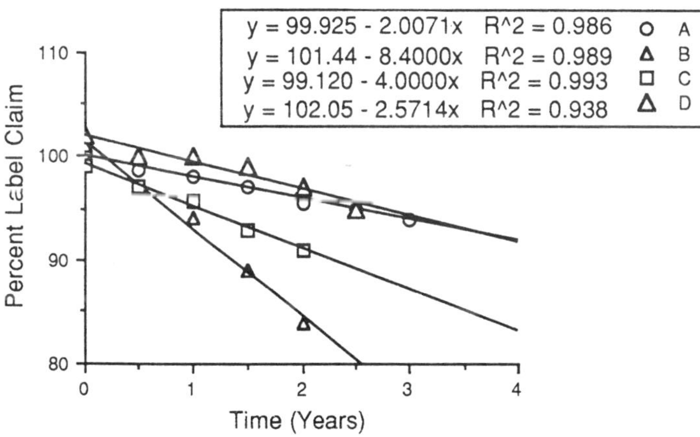

Figure 5.2 Data from Table 5.2 presented graphically without modification. The least squares fits are shown in the figure.

[7]Strictly speaking, this is only correct if the initial data points are all close to the same value (as is the case here).

[8]Any fractional time may be used. For solution work, it is often more convenient to use $t_{1/2}$.

TABLE 5.3. Data for the Decomposition of a Drug in a Solid Dosage Form.

Time (Years)	Fraction of Label Claim			
	Batch A	Batch B	Batch C	Batch D
0	1.0	1.0	1.0	102
0.5	0.98	0.96	0.98	0.98
1.0	0.98	0.933	0.966	0.98
1.5	0.97	0.881	0.939	0.971
2.0	0.955	0.832	0.919	0.951
2.5	95			0.931
3.0	94			

or

$$t_{90} = 0.09825/2.0051 = 0.049 \tag{5.9}$$

If the data in Table 5.3 are expressed in reduced time,[9] then the data in Table 5.4 result, and these data are presented graphically in Figure 5.4. The advantage of such plotting is that (a) it shows *all* the data in an easy-to-read fashion and (b) it demonstrates the kinetic mode, i.e., whether linear or curved.

In the case where first-order is suspected, the procedure is the same, except that the fractional life is obtained by a plot of ln [Fraction] versus time, and for, e.g., t_{90}

$$\ln [0.9] = -kt_{90} \tag{5.10}$$

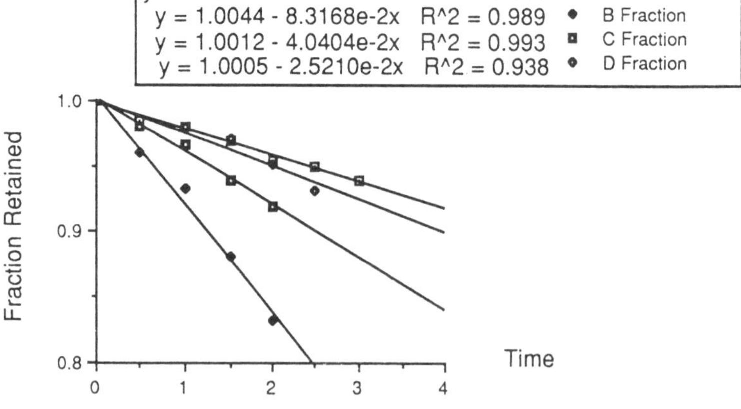

Figure 5.3 Data in Figure 5.3 expressed as fraction retained.

[9]The treatment is strictly correct with logarithmic data.

TABLE 5.4. Data from Table 5.3 Expressed in Reduced Parameters.

Time/t_{90}	Batch A t_{90}=4.90	Batch B t_{90}=1.256	Batch C t_{90}=2.478	Batch D t_{90}=3.987
0	1.000			
0.102	0.980			
0.204	0.980			
0.308	0.970			
0.408	0.954			
0.51	0.949			
0.612	0.939			
0		1.000		
0.398		0.960		
0.796		0.933		
1.194		0.881		
1.592		0.832		
0			1.000	
0.202			0.980	
0.404			0.966	
0.605			0.939	
0.807			0.919	
0				1.000
0.125				0.980
0.251				0.980
0.376				0.971
0.502				0.951
0.627				0.931

5.6 COMMON CONSIDERATIONS

After having discussed presentation mode, e.g., in reduced parameter format, the next question that arises is what type of curve-fitting one should attempt. The kinetic data in Table 5.5 are an example of this. Most chemists are aware of the importance of the order of a reaction, but let us assume that the data are approached from a zero data and experience base.

If one considers a series of data points, the first consideration is, in general, to take into consideration the shape of the curve and seek a function with which to fit the data, a function that is consistent with the "limits" of the curve.

Given the points in Table 5.5, one might plot these and obtain a graph of the type shown in Figure 5.5. The best fit is shown in the caption, and it would seem that it would be quite good. However, if the data are simply

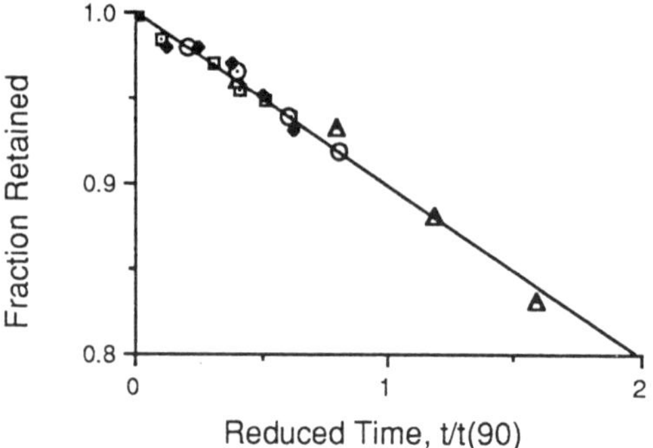

Figure 5.4 Data from Table 5.4. Data are plotted using fraction retained and reduced time (t/t_{90}). Legend: A = squares, B = triangles, C = circles, and D = diamonds. The least squares fit is for all the fractions combined and is $y = 1.0007 - 0.10135x$ ($R^2 = 0.986$).

plotted and the chord drawn between the extreme points, it is obvious that *all* the points are below the chord and that, therefore, there is *curvature.*

The second point to consider is that, most often, a scientist has some idea of what the functionality is. Given, for instance, the data in Figure 5.5, a chemist would automatically, as a first thought, consider treating them by a first-order reaction equation (Figure 5.6). As a second thought, he might think of considering them a first-order reaction with equilibrium conditions, and as a third thought, he might consider them to be a second-order reaction. However, in many such situations, practitioners simply consider the first option, arguing that the fit (in Figure 5.5) is good, so why worry about it.

If the data in the first two columns of Table 5.5 are treated in a first-order fashion, i.e., by

TABLE 5.5. Fraction of Potency Retained as a Function of Time.

Time	Fraction Retained C/C_0	$\ln[C/C_0]$	$\hat{C/C_0}$ (Eq. 5.13)
0	1.0	0	1.0
10	0.90	-0.105	0.902
20	0.82	-0.198	0.817
30	0.74	-0.301	0.739
40	0.66	-0.416	0.669
50	0.61	-0.494	0.606
60	0.55	-0.598	0.549

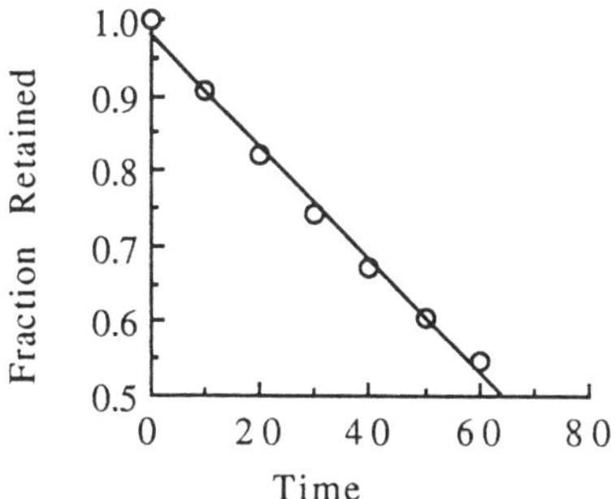

Figure 5.5 Best fit. $y = 0.981 - 0.0075x$ ($R^2 = 0.99$).

$$\ln [C/C_0] = -k_1 t \tag{5.11}$$

then good linearity results, as shown in Figure 5.7.

It should be pointed out that, if a "best" fit is found by a so-called transformation, e.g., in the above case,

$$\ln [C/C_0] = -0.00303 - 0.0099587t \tag{5.12}$$

then it is a good practice to show the data in "Cartesian" presentation, i.e., in the above case as

$$[C/C_0] = 0.997e^{-0.00996t} \tag{5.13}$$

To do this, lacking more sophisticated programs, one might simply write a program in BASIC as shown in Table 5.6.

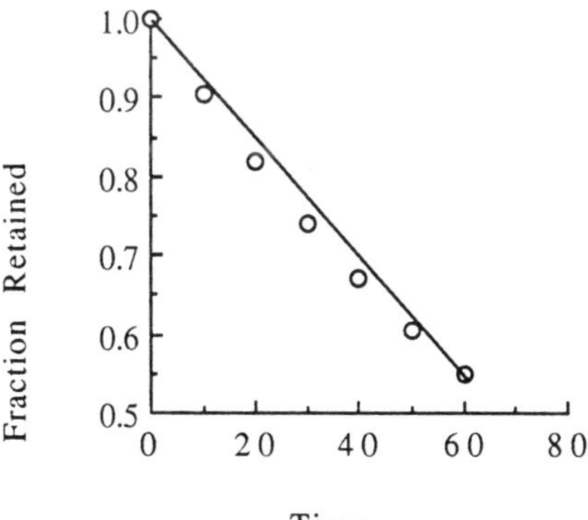

Figure 5.6 Data from Table 5.5.

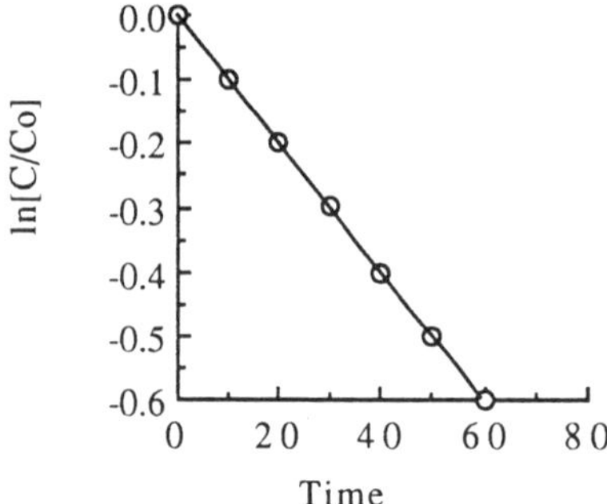

Figure 5.7 Data from Table 5.5 treated by Equation (5.11).

With some primers, command 120 should be LPRINT T,X1. In general, dot-matrix printers are used for the results printout. This would be as shown in Table 5.5, last column. The last two columns would be plotted versus time in a CricketGraph™. To show the "theoretical" curve, the points on the fitted curve (denoted by ^) are changed from symbols to points, and the fit by "interpolation" applied. The equation for the curve would be added by means of the tools, resulting in Figure 5.8. It is noted that the curve appears as a "curve," and the points (the experimental points) remain as points.

It will become apparent later why it is important to present the data in "untransformed" mode (Figure 5.8), rather than in "transformed" mode (Figure 5.7).

5.7 GENERAL CURVE FORMS

It is seen in the writing above, that the selection of the equation form often is based on "knowledge" in the area, but at the onset, we shall simply assume no such knowledge. It will be assumed that data points exist and that, as a first approximation, we want to fit the data to a curve and find an equation for the curve. To this end, it is advantageous to know what the equations are for several common types of curves.

TABLE 5.6. Program for Generating Data from Equation (5.13).

```
100  FOR T = 0 TO 60 STEP 10
110  X1 = 0.997*EXP(-0.00996*T)
120  PRINT T,X1
130  NEXT T
```

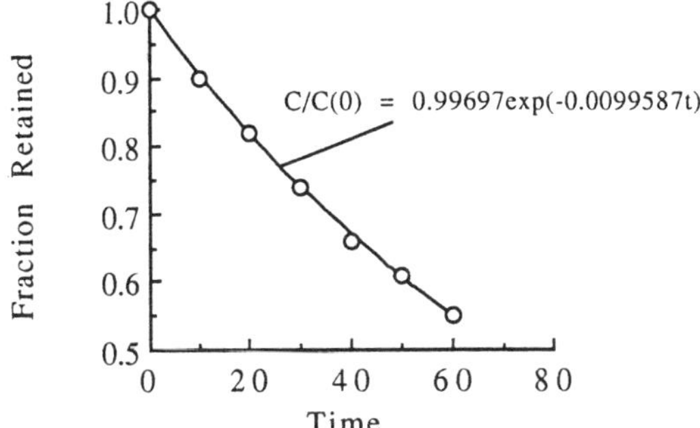

Figure 5.8 Data from last column in Table 5.5.

5.8 SECOND-ORDER CURVE, FIRST-ORDER CURVE WITH EQUILIBRIUM

A second-order curve and a first-order curve with equilibrium have the shape shown in Figure 5.9.

The equation for this can be of several types:

(A)
$$\ln [y_\infty - y] = -kt + \ln [y_\infty] \tag{5.14}$$

or

$$y = y_\infty[1 - e^{-kt}] \tag{5.15}$$

(B)
$$\ln [y/(1 - y)] = -kt \qquad 1 > y > 0 \tag{5.16}$$

The latter case is an example of the situation where there is a zero-time, or zero-point, lack of definition. This is often the case in curve-fitting and

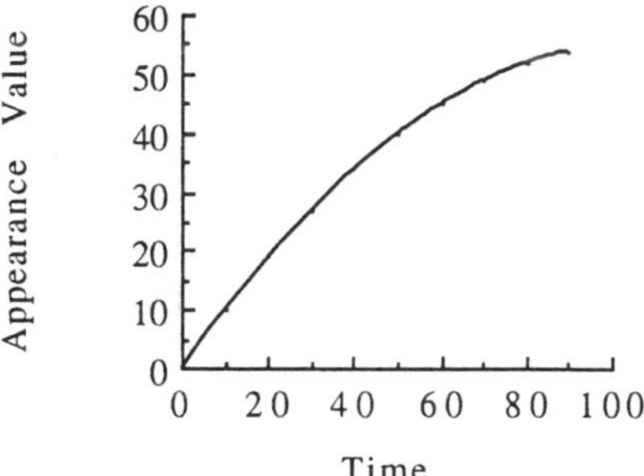

Figure 5.9 Second-order curve.

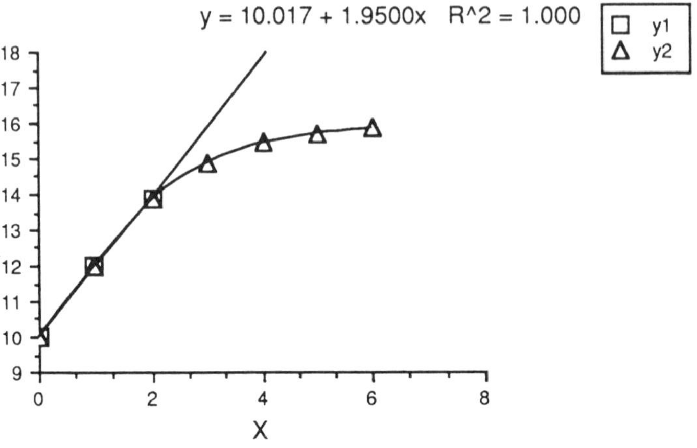

Figure 5.10 Data in Table 5.7 plotted on ordinary Cartesian graph paper.

modelistic situations. A famous case is the Gibbs isotherm in surface chemistry.

5.9 THE SIGMA-MINUS PLOT

As mentioned, the first attempt at organizing data is often to plot them. It is possible at the onset ($x = 0,1,2$) that the assumption of simple linearity ($y1$) prevails, but as more y-values become available ($y2$), it is apparent from Figure 5.10 that linearity is lost.

Often, as shown in Table 5.7 and Figure 5.10, the curvature is such that it tends toward an asymptote, in this case $y = 16$. If the differences between 16 and the y-values are plotted, then their logarithms form a straight line, i.e.,

$$\ln [16 - y] = -kt + A \tag{5.17}$$

Note that A should be given by

$$A = \ln [16] \tag{5.18}$$

TABLE 5.7. Two Simple Data Sets Chosen for Curve Fitting.

x or t	0	1	2	3	4	5	6
y	10	12	13.9				
y 2	10	1 2	13.9	14.9	15.45	15.72	15.86

TABLE 5.8. Two Simple Data Sets Chosen for Curve Fitting.

x	0	1	2	3	4	5	8
y 2	10	12	13.9	14.9	15.45	15.72	15.86
16-y2	6	4	2.1	1.1	0.55	0.28	0.14

if the line applies over the entire domain. To test for this in a simultaneous fashion, the two equations might be combined to read

$$\ln [1 - (y/16)] = -kt \tag{5.19}$$

If the line does not go through the origin, then amendment is made by either introducing a lag time, t_i, or denoting the asymptote, y_∞:

$$\ln [1 - (y/y_\infty)] = -k[t - t_i] \tag{5.20}$$

This is correct if the intersection with $y = 0$ is at positive x. If it is at negative x, then the equation becomes

$$\ln [1 - (y/y_\infty)] = A - kt \tag{5.21}$$

and some initial value is assigned to the dependent variable. The latter is obviously the case in Table 5.8 and Figure 5.11. Here, ln [16] = 2.77, and the line obtains this value at negative x-values.

The technique, in different variations, is often referred to as stripping, feathering, or sigma-minus plotting. The notation "sigma-minus" stems from sigma denoting differences, and the minus means that they are

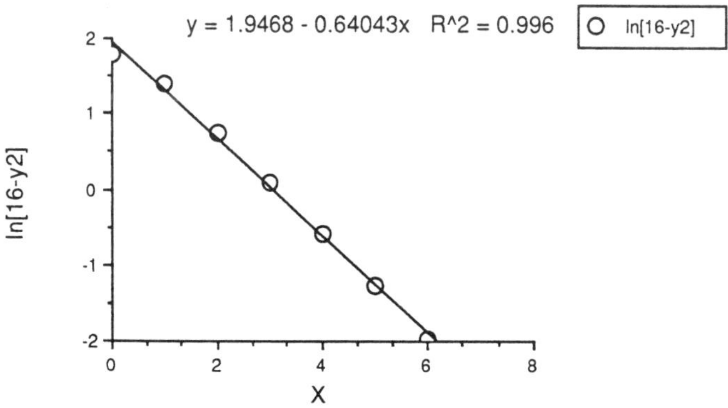

Figure 5.11 Data from Table 5.7 treated by sigma-minus plotting.

measured from the asymptote down to the curve. Examples of sigma-minus situations are (a) dissolution beyond the sink conditions (approximately) and (b) equilibration of a sample at a given relative humidity (approximately).

5.10 THE LOGARITHMIC PLOT

It is often said that anything may be linearized by taking logarithms. That this is not so is demonstrated in Figure 5.12, where the data from Table 5.8 have been plotted in this fashion, i.e.,

$$\ln [y2] = a + b \ln [x] \tag{5.22}$$

where a and b are constants.

The logarithmic relation is often considered in dimensionless analysis, which shall be touched upon later.

5.11 POLYNOMIAL PLOTS

It will be demonstrated later that polynomial fitting is often done by multiple regression. If such regressions are performed on the data in Table 5.8, then it would appear that a third-order polynomial gives quite a good fit. This is shown in Figure 5.13.

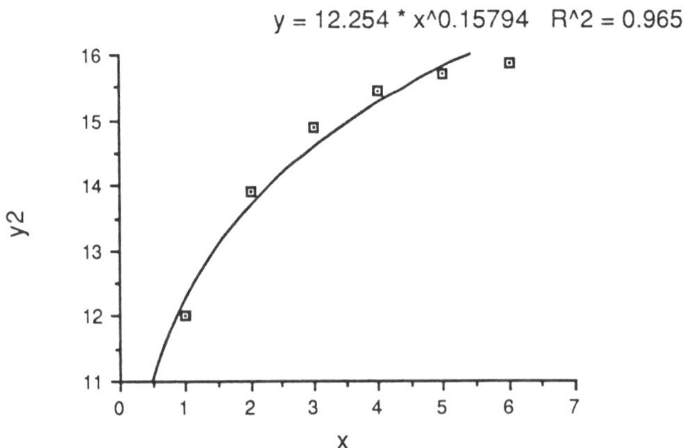

Figure 5.12 Data from Table 5.8 plotted according to Equation (5.22).

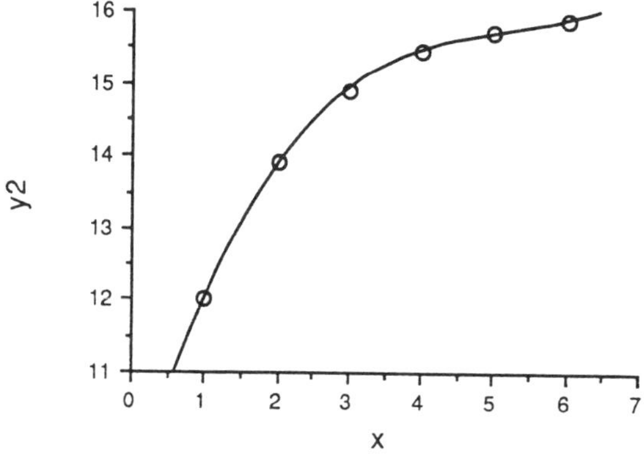

Figure 5.13 The data in Table 5.8 treated by a polynomial approximation.

5.12 INVERSE PLOTS

Often, data give the impression that the variables might be inversely related, i.e.,

$$(1/y) = (a/x) + b \tag{5.23}$$

Linear plotting in this fashion is dangerous, as shown in the following. To demonstrate this, the program in Table 5.9 is written to generate values that truly follow Equation (5.23) or, rather, the variant:

$$y = x/(b + ax) \tag{5.24}$$

The data treatment as shown in Table 5.9 will result in the graph in Figure 5.14; a and b are constants.

If one sets $a = 1$ and $b = 2$, one obtains the values in Table 5.10 to four significant figures. The last column has the theoretical y-values perturbed ever so slightly (to the point one might expect experimentally). The data

TABLE 5.9. Data That Might Be Inversely Related.

x	y	1/x	1/y
1	12.5	1	0.08
2	16.67	0.5	0.06
3	17.5	0.3333	0.057
4	18.75	0.25	0.053
5	19.33	0.2	0.0517
6	19.67	0.1666	0.0508

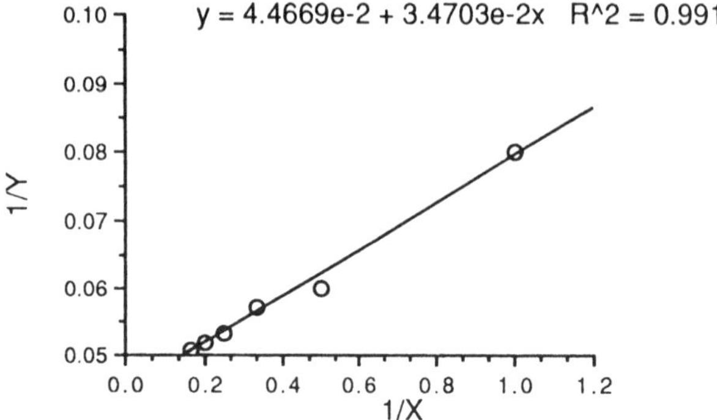

Figure 5.14 Data from Table 5.10 treated in inverse fashion.

are plotted in inverse fashion in Figure 5.14. It is noted that the extracted a-value is 7% too low, and the b-value is 6% too high.

The data seem to fit fairly well, but it is incorrect to judge the goodness of fit from the transformed curve. A curve of the type in Equation (5.24) is generated using $a = 0.034703$ and $b = 0.04669$ (the values from Figure 5.14) in the program in Table 5.9. The results are as shown in Table 5.11.

When these data are plotted versus the experimental data from Table 5.9, then Figure 5.15 results. It is quite obvious that, although the fit in Equation (5.14) seemed quite good, when presented as $y = f(x)$, there is quite a bias.

If the data are introduced into SigmaPlot®, then the curve fitting is as shown in Table 5.12. Executing the program then gives the output in Table

TABLE 5.10. Program for Generating Curves from Parameter Values.

```
100 PRINT "Inverse Plot"
110 INPUT "Number of Steps="; N
120 INPUT "Highest X-value="; X1
130 INPUT "Smallest X-value="; X2
140 INPUT "Parameter A="; A
150 INPUT "Parameter B="'; B
200 Z = (X1-X2)/N
210 FOR T = X1 TO X2 STEP Z
220 Y = T/(B+A*T)
230 PRINT T, Y
240 NEXT X1
```

TABLE 5.11. Output for Program in Table 5.10 Using $A = 0.034703$ and $B = 0.044669$.

x	y
1	12.60
2	12.53
3	20.16
4	21.80
5	22.92
6	23.73

5.13. The last column gives information as to whether there is dependency[10] between the parameters and a number close to unity would so indicate, as opposed to this case. Placing the parameter values in column 3 and the $y\sim$-values in column 4 then results in Table 5.14.

These data are graphed in Figure 5.16, and it is obvious that the fit of $y = f(x)$ is good, so it is obvious that the nonlinear regression is better than the approximate methods.

5.13 DEDUCTION AND CURVE FITTING

Often, curves go through maxima, and it is of importance to consider the situation in a phenomenological sense and even to think of the data in

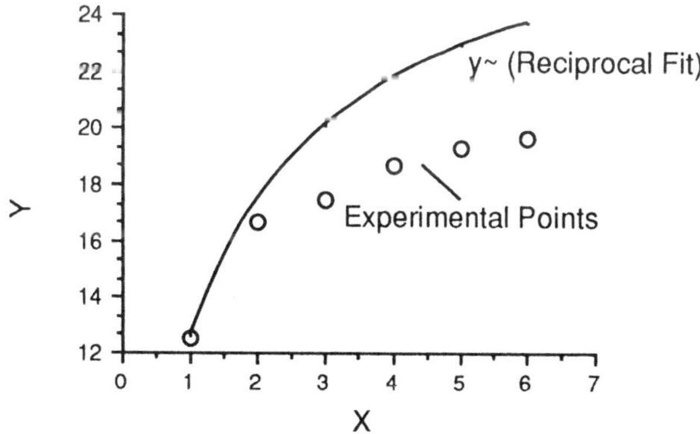

Figure 5.15 Data from Tables 5.9 and 5.11.

[10]Dependency = (variance of the parameter, other parameters constant) divided by (variance of the parameter, other parameters changing). SigmaPlot® gives this value. If it is close to unity, then there is dependence between the parameters.

TABLE 5.12. Function Input into SigmaPlot®.

```
[Parameters]
A = 1.52
B = 2.31
[Variables]
x = col(1)
y = col(2)
[Equations]
f=(x/(A+B*x))
[Constraints]
A>0
B>0
[Options]
Iterations = 100
stepsize = 1
tolerance = 0.01
```

TABLE 5.13. Output from SigmaPlot® Program in Table 5.12.

Converged, tolerance satisfied

Norm: 0.615781

Parameter	Value	St.Er.	CV(%)	Dependency
A	3.353e-02	2.175e-03	6.487e+00	0.721019
B	4.507e-02	7.477e-04	1.657e+00	0.721019

TABLE 5.14. Output from SigmaPlot® Program in Table 5.12.

x	y	A,B	y~
1	12.5	0.033529	12.722
2	16.67	0.045073	16.172
3	17.5		17.778
4	18.75		18.707
5	19.33		19.313
6	19.67		19.739

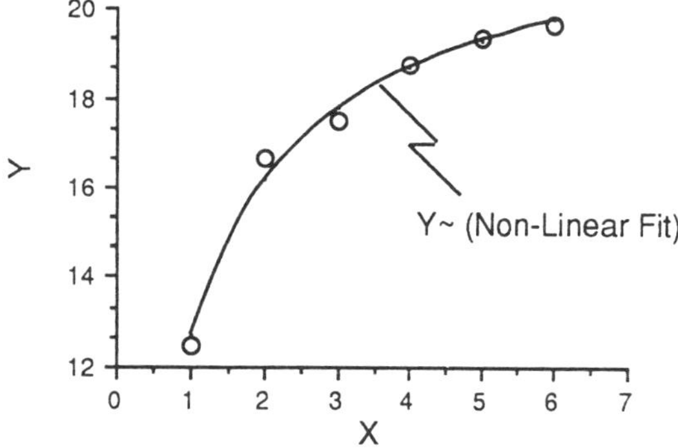

Figure 5.16 Data from the nonlinear fitting mode in Tables 5.12 to 5.14.

a modelistic sense, i.e., what is giving rise to the maximum. This type of deduction often leads to direct modeling.

It is also, often, the case that one desires to curve-fit data reported in literature to a given type of equation system, and if it is assumed that the data one is desirous of treating have the shape in Figure 5.17, what would be the best approach?

The best method for converting a curve into a set of data is to contact the author of the data and ask if raw data are available. If the publication is based on a Ph.D. thesis, then the data are obtained from the source library. But often, these methods are not available, and in such a case, it is simplest to paste a 1 cm square piece of transparent graph paper over the curve, and note each point in graph paper units. These are then converted to actual units by recording the axis scales as well. From Figure 5.17, the set in Table 5.15 is derived.

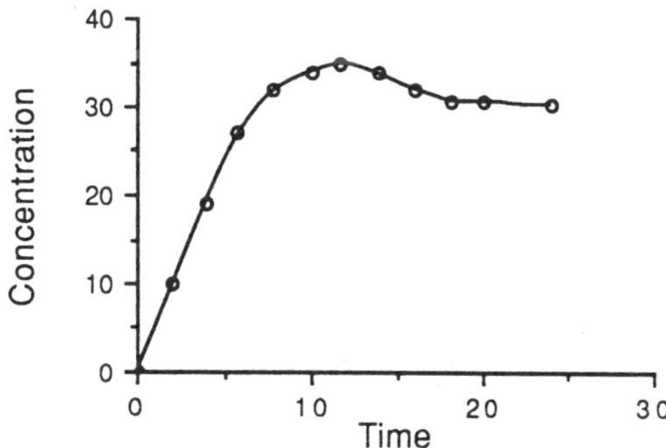

Figure 5.17 Dissolution curve of a metastable polymorph.

TABLE 5.15. Data Obtained from Figure 5.17.

Time (t)	Concentration (C)
0	0
2.0	10
3.8	19
5.7	27
7.8	32
10	34
11.6	35
13.8	34
16	32
18	30.8
20	30.6
24	30.4

It is possible to simply fit this, e.g., to a third-order polynomial, and this is done in Figure 5.18.

The problem is that the domain of the function is from $t = 0$ to $t =$ infinity, and the "upswing" after 25 minutes is unrealistic. It is possible to say, however, that the function is valid up to $t = 20$, but this is a restriction.

If the data are presented in this manner, it is better, rather than using the curve that the computer generates, to generate numbers for the curve and simply draw it in (using Interpolate on the CricketGraph™ address) and the domain to which it is confined.

The third-order curve in Figure 5.18 is

$$y = -1.2265 + 7.2355x - 0.46485x^2 + 0.0090857x^3 \quad (5.25)$$

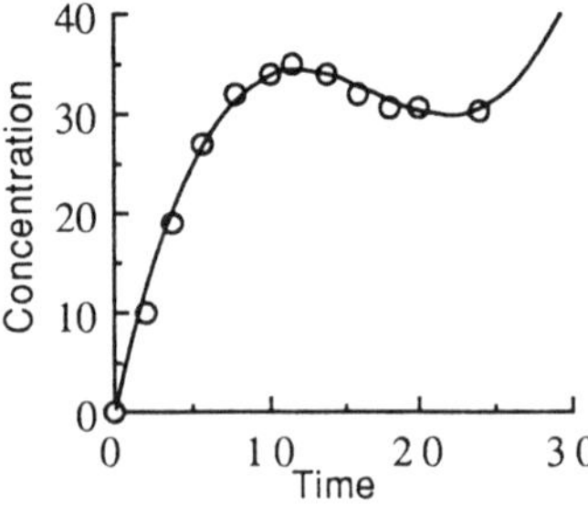

Figure 5.18 Data from Table 5.15 fitted to a third-order polynomial.

TABLE 5.16. Data Generator for Equation (5.25).

```
100 FOR X = 0 TO 25 STEP 5
110 Y1 = -1.2265 + 7.2355*X
120 Y2 = -0.46485*(X^2) + 0.0090857*(x^3)
130 Y3 = Y1 + y2
140 PRINT X,Y3
150 NEXT X
```

Points fitting this equation can be generated, most easily by computer, e.g., by the program listed in Table 5.16 (in BASIC). And, again, the note is made that LPRINT may have to be used rather than PRINT. In running the program, the numbers in Table 5.17 result.

These results are then entered as a third column in the graphics program (in this case, CricketGraph™). The symbol for the data in Table 5.17 are made a point, and the experimental points are left as a given symbol, e.g., an open circle. The curve through the points (not the circles) is drawn by means of *Interpolate* under the *Curve Fit* address. The result of this is shown in Figure 5.19.

5.14 ARE THE DATA MONOPHASIC OR BIPHASIC?

It is, of course, not necessary that the curve is a result of one process, and if it is a result of two or more, then the domain should be divided up into such domains where appropriate fitting can be done.

It is also noted that, in curve-fitting, it is not necessary to be concerned about what the actual physical phenomenon is. If one considers the process to be biphasic, then the first part of the data in Table 5.15 is fit to be a parabola, as shown in Figure 5.20.

TABLE 5.17. Printout from Table 5.14.

X	Y3
0	-1.23
5	24.47
10	33.73
15	33.38
20	30.23
25	31.1

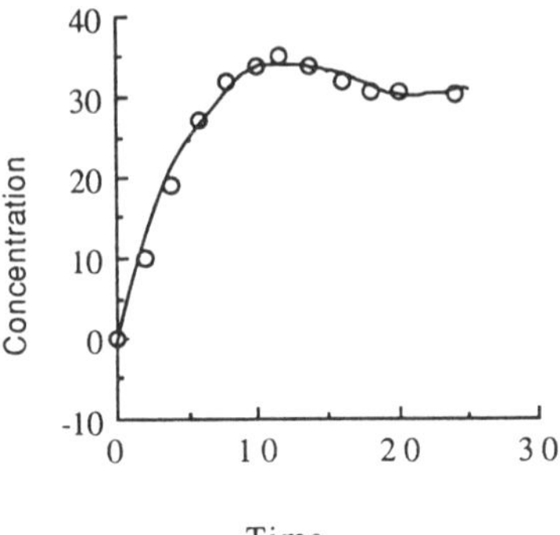

Figure 5.19 Experimental data from Table 5.14 fitted by curve in Table 5.15.

The best parabola (from CricketGraph™) is given by

$$y = -0.60499 + 6.3422x - 0.28426x^2 \tag{5.26}$$

It is noted that the maximum in the curve is given by

$$dy/dx = 6.342 - 0.0568x \tag{5.27}$$

i.e., the maximum is at

$$x = 6.342/0.0568 = 11.18 \tag{5.28}$$

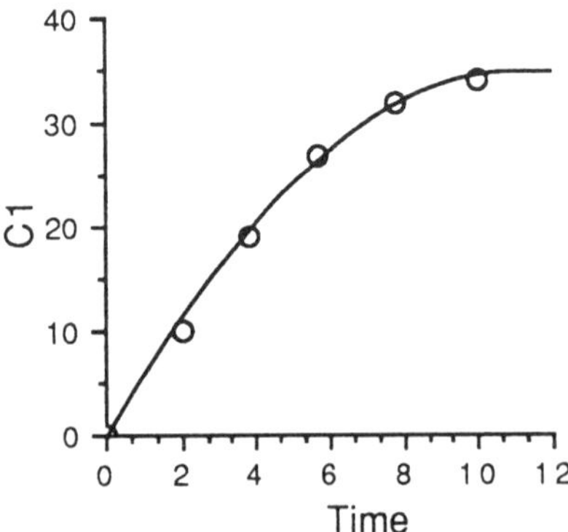

Figure 5.20 The first points from Table 5.15 (below 10 minutes) are fitted to a parabola: $y = -0.60499 + 6.3422x - 0.28426x^2$ ($R^2 = 0.998$).

At this point, the y value is

$$y = -0.605 + 70.90 - 35.50 = 34.80 \tag{5.29}$$

For the second part, the curve must (a) have a value of 34.80 at $x = 11.18$, (b) have a slope of zero at $x = 11.18$, and (c) must asymptote at $x \rightarrow \infty$ at (estimated) $y = 30$.

The problem here is that this part of the curve cannot be a simple sigma-minus type plot, because of condition (b). A better fitting function would be like a normal error curve:[11]

$$C = 30 + (34.8 - 30)\exp(-k(t - 11.18)^2) \tag{5.30}$$

The problem then is to find k. It follows from the above that

$$\ln[(C - 30)/4.8] = -k(t - 11.18)^2 \tag{5.31}$$

The transformed variables are introduced into CricketGraph™ (or a similar program), or the plotting is done by hand. The best fit for this line is

$$y = -0.050717 - 0.037375x \tag{5.32}$$

This is *not* all that good, and some refinement could probably be made (e.g., by iterating the preexponential value and the asymptote value, e.g., to 30.3 and 4.5). Accepting the above as a first estimate, however, the second part of the curve would be of the form

$$C = 30 + 4.5\exp[-0.0374(x - 11.18)^2] \qquad 11.18 < t < \infty \tag{5.33}$$

The values for C at the time points above 11.18 are shown in Table 5.18 and are plotted in Figure 5.21.

TABLE 5.18. Values of C for Times above 11.18.

Time	Experimental Value	Fitted Value
11.6	35	34.7
13.8	34	33.8
16	32	32.2
18	30.8	31.1
20	30.6	30.5

[11]This will be discussed further in the following chapter.

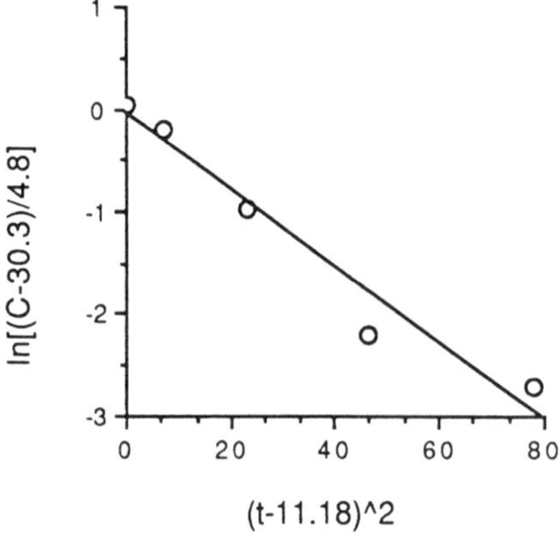

Figure 5.21 Data fitted to Equation (5.33): $y = -0.050717 - 0.037375x$ ($R^2 = 0.957$).

It is noted that there are many programs that "curve-fit" data, but one must look carefully for the features of the curve, and let the functions used assume the correct values at the boundaries and at optima. The full curve is shown in Figure 5.22. It is seen, then, that there is, at times, logic in considering data as being biphasic.

5.15 CURVE-FITTING THE NORMALIZED FREQUENCY FUNCTION

A great deal of attention will be given to the normal error curve and normally distributed data in the next chapter, but an introduction into these is appropriate at this point.

When large numbers of data (X) are accumulated, they are often presented in histogram form; i.e., the data are split up into intervals (Δ) of the

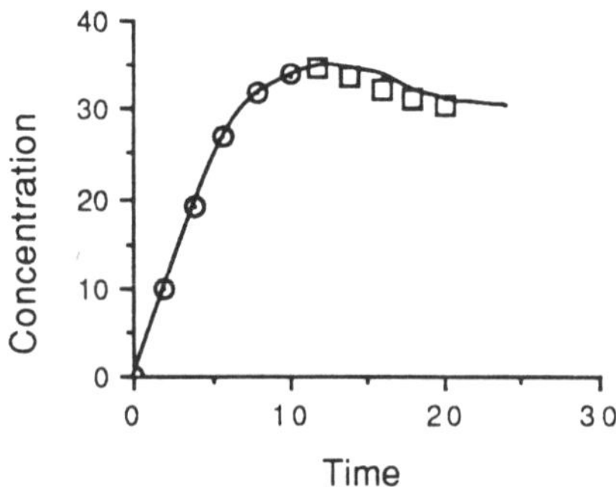

Figure 5.22 Data from Figure 5.20 and Table 5.18 combined.

variable, and the number of occurrences (N_i) in each interval are recorded. These data are often converted into frequencies (by dividing N_i in each interval with the total number of data, N).

The average (X_{avg}) and standard deviation, σ, of the numbers are calculated, and the unit of the x-axis chosen as

$$x = (X - X_{avg})/\sigma \tag{5.34}$$

If the frequency curve is normalized by making the area under it equal to unity, then the so-called Gaussian frequency curve is obtained. This will have the shape shown in Figure 5.23. The curve is symmetric and has two inflection points. It is noted that at the point of inflection, $x = 1$.

The question is, from a phenomenological point of view, what would a "good" equation be for this curve? One can arrive at this equation by phenomenological deduction.

The features of the curve are

(1) It is symmetric, i.e., $y = f(a) = f(-a)$.
(2) It tails off asymptotically to zero if x goes to either $\pm\infty$.

Here f denotes "function of." The strategy is to find a function that has these qualities. There are several functions that will tail off at zero when x goes to infinity, e.g.,

$$y = \exp(-kx) \tag{5.35}$$

and

$$y = (1/kx) \tag{5.36}$$

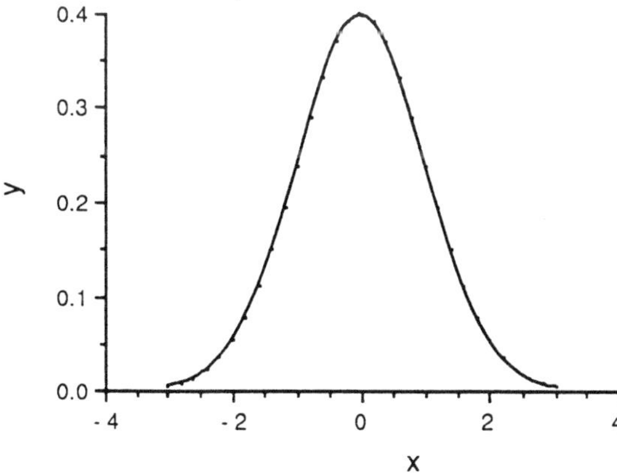

Figure 5.23 Shape of a normal frequency curve.

TABLE 5.19. Dissolution Data.

Time	% Dissolved	Z
0	0	
5	1	-2.33
10	10	-1.28
20	60	0.26
25	82	0.92
30	94	1.555
45	97	1.88

Data are often of a normally or log-normally distributed nature and, for this reason, are plotted on probability paper. The problem with simply plotting on such paper is that an equation cannot be arrived at.

To this end, use is made of the normal error curve, Appendix 1. The appendix is tabulated in such a way that it is easy to find the area corresponding to a given Z-value and also easy to find a Z-value corresponding to a certain area.

It is instructive to consider such a case, and the one chosen here is the case of Wagner (1969) who suggested that dissolution curves of tablets be treated as log-normal in time. An example of how this is done is shown in Table 5.19. The data from the first two columns are plotted in Figure 5.24.

The data in the second column are converted by means of Appendix 2 to "Z-values"; i.e., the normal standard deviate value, *Z*, is found, for which the area under the normal error curve corresponds to the cumulative frequency. This gives rise to column 3, and the data are plotted in this fashion versus the logarithm of time, and the graph in Figure 5.25 results.

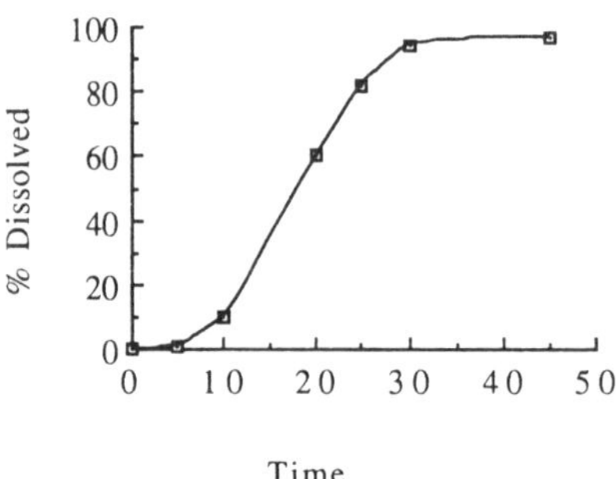

Figure 5.24 Data from Table 5.19.

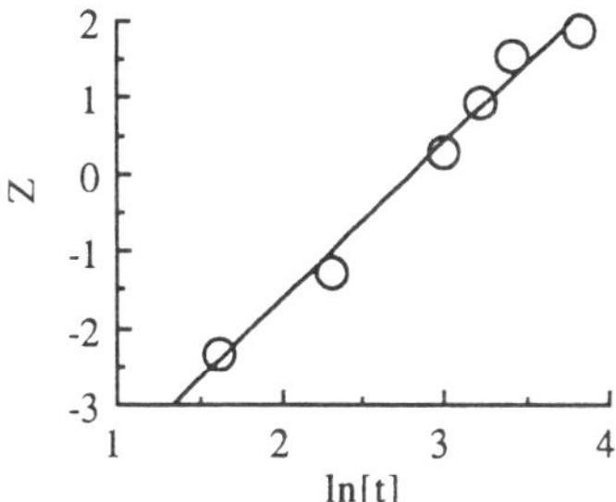

Figure 5.25 Data from Table 5.16.

5.17 WEIBULL PLOTTING

There are cases where distribution data are best treated by the so-called Weibull function given by

$$\ln\{-\ln(y)\} = -k(x - x_i) \tag{5.52}$$

where y is cumulative frequency. The manner in which this is done is left as an exercise for the reader in Problem 5.1.

5.18 PROBLEMS

(1) The data in Figure 5.26 have been taken out of recent literature and deal with the rate of transformation of a metastable polymorph into a stable modification of a particulate solid, which may be considered monodisperse.

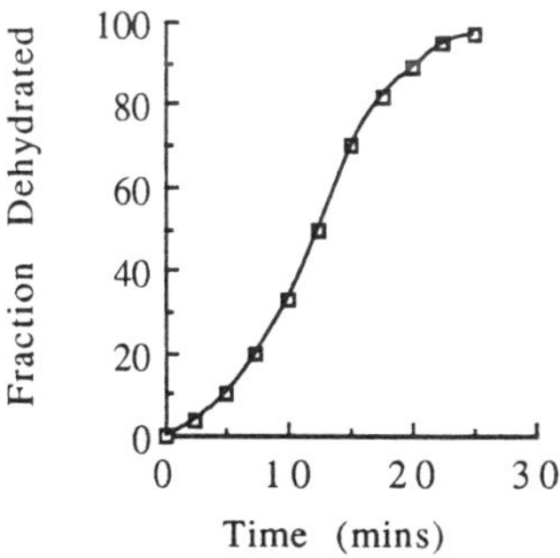

Figure 5.26 Transformation data.

Is it possible to postulate that the transformation occurs because of the following:

- There first has to be created a nucleus in the individual particle?
- Once this nucleus is formed, the transformation of that particular particle is instantaneous?

(Hint: Assume the times of nucleation to be normally distributed, and check to see if the data "plot" as a normal distribution function. For example, what is the average nucleation time, and what is the standard deviation?)

(2) The function

$$y = A\exp(-(x_e - x_{(e)\text{avg}})^4/\{q\sigma^4\}) \tag{5.53}$$

is, from a curve-fitting point of view a suitable candidate to describe normally distributed data. x_e is the experimental value.

Use the assumption that the inflection point is at ± 1 standard deviation from the mean, and derive q and A. In deriving the value of the normalization integral, describe how you arrived at the value of the gamma function you used. The gamma function is

$$\Gamma(z) = \int_0^\infty u^{z-1}e^{-u}du \tag{5.54}$$

Note that

$$\Gamma(z + 1) = z! \tag{5.55}$$

$$\Gamma(1/2) = \sqrt{\pi} \tag{5.56}$$

and

$$\Gamma(z + 1) = z\Gamma(z) \tag{5.57}$$

(3) Averages are distributed by the student t-distribution, which shall be discussed in a later chapter. The values of t are shown in Appendix 3. In programs for least squares fitting in BASIC, it is convenient to find an adequate curve (a curve-fit equation) to be utilized for the value of student t in a program for $63 > N > 7$, for instance, a step sequence like the one shown in Table 5.20.

In this manner, if N is between 7 and 63, an approximation function would be used, and if $N > 63$, then it is simply assumed to be constant (a

TABLE 5.20. Program to Fit the Student *t*-Function.

```
991 IF N2 > 7 GOTO 992
992 IF N2 > 63 GOTO 996
994 T =
996 T = 1.96
```

good approximation). For $N < 7$, the individual *t*-values are inserted in the program.

The alternative to this would be to list sixty-three *t*-values.

(4) Wagner (1969) suggested that dissolution curves of tablets or capsules could be treated as log-normal (percent probit versus log time). Treat the data in Table 5.21 in this fashion. [The data have been reconstructed from data dealing with dissolution of aspirin tablets, published by Javaid and Cadwallader (1972)]. The data have been amplified for the purpose of demonstrating data treatment.

Treat the data as suggested by Wagner (1969). Some authors (Lippmann, 1972) have suggested using a Weibull function for this. Plot the data in Weibull fashion. Which presentation mode is best, log normal or Weibull? What criterion should be used for this comparison? In inspecting the graphs, what conclusion can be reached regarding the presentation modes?

5.19 ANSWERS

(1) The data are read off the graph in Figure 5.26, and the first two col-

TABLE 5.21. Dissolution Data.

Time	% Dissolved
0	0
1	4
2	10
4	26.3
6	40
8	49.6
10	58
12	66.2
16	77.1
20	85
25	89.9

TABLE 5.22. Data from Figure 5.26 and Their Weibull Transformation.

Time (min)	x	ln{-ln[x]}
2.5	0.020	1.364
5	0.100	0.834
7.5	0.210	0.445
10	0.330	0.103
12.5	0.500	-0.367
15	0.700	-1.031
17.5	0.800	-1.500
20	0.860	-1.892

umns in Table 5.22 are constructed. The x-values are then converted to ln $[x]$ (which are all negative) and then to $-\ln[x]$ (which are all positive), and the logarithm of this latter is then obtained and placed in column 3. These data are then plotted in Figure 5.27, and as seen, the Weibull transformation linearizes the data.

(2) For convenience, the variable

$$x = (x_e - x_{(e)\text{avg}}) \tag{5.58}$$

is used, so that the function is

$$(1/A)y = e^{-x^4/q\sigma^4} \tag{5.59}$$

The second derivative of this function is

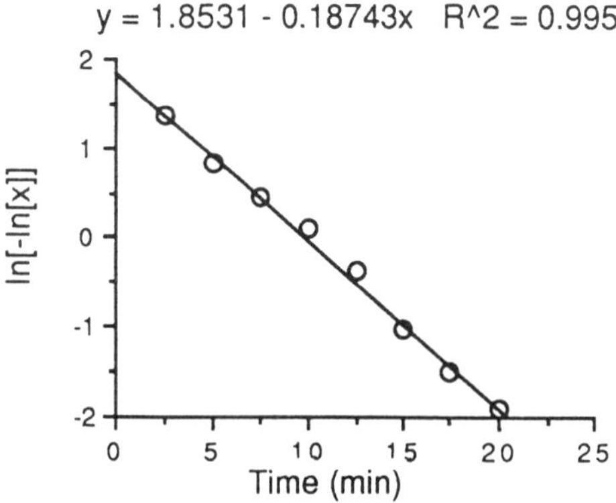

Figure 5.27 Data from Table 5.22.

$$(1/A)d^2y/dx^2 = e^{-x^4/q\sigma^4}/(q\sigma^4)[-12x^2 + (16x^6/q\sigma^4)] \quad (5.60)$$

which equals zero when $x = \sigma$, i.e.,

$$q = (16/12) = 1.33 \quad (5.61)$$

Normalization requires that

$$A\int_{-\infty}^{\infty} e^{-x^4/1.3\sigma^4}dx = 2A \qquad \int_{0}^{\infty} e^{-x^4/1.3\sigma^4}dx = 1 \quad (5.62)$$

the first equality arising from the symmetry condition.

We now use the substitution

$$u = x^4/1.3\sigma^4 \quad (5.63)$$

i.e.,

$$x = (u1.3\sigma^4)^{1/4} \quad (5.64)$$

It follows from Equations (5.63) and (5.64) that

$$du = 4x^3/(1.3\sigma^4)dx = 4(1.3\sigma^4)^{-1/4}u^{3/4}dx \quad (5.65)$$

So that the integral in Equation (5.62) becomes

$$0.25 \times (1.3^{1/4} \times \sigma\int_{0}^{\infty} u^{-3/4}e^{-u}du = 1 \quad (5.66)$$

The integral is the gamma function evaluated at 1/4. Although this may be obtained from tables, it is noted from Equation (5.57) that

$$\Gamma(0.25 + 1) = 0.25\Gamma(0.25) \quad (5.67)$$

i.e.,

$$\Gamma(0.25) = 4\Gamma(1.25) \quad (5.68)$$

TABLE 5.23. Values of the Gamma Function.

x	0.5	1	1.5	2	3	4
Γ(x)	1.77	1	0.885	1	2	3

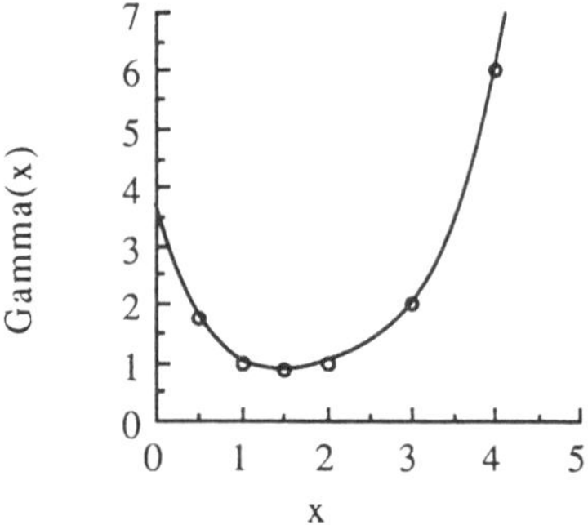

Figure 5.28 Graph of gamma function ($R^2 = 1$).

If a table were not available, the value of $\Gamma(1.25)$ could be evaluated by curve fitting. The values of the gamma function from 0.5 to 4 are listed in Table 5.23. These data are plotted in Figure 5.28.

The best (polynomial) fit of these data is

$$\Gamma(x) = 3.7021 - 5.5383x - 3.9083x^2 - 1.2170x^3 + 0.1555x^4 \tag{5.69}$$

When $x = 1.25$ is inserted into this, the value of

$$\Gamma(1.25) = 0.8886292 \tag{5.70}$$

is obtained. Hence [Equation (5.58)],

$$\Gamma(0.25) = 4 \times 0.889 = 3.555 \tag{5.71}$$

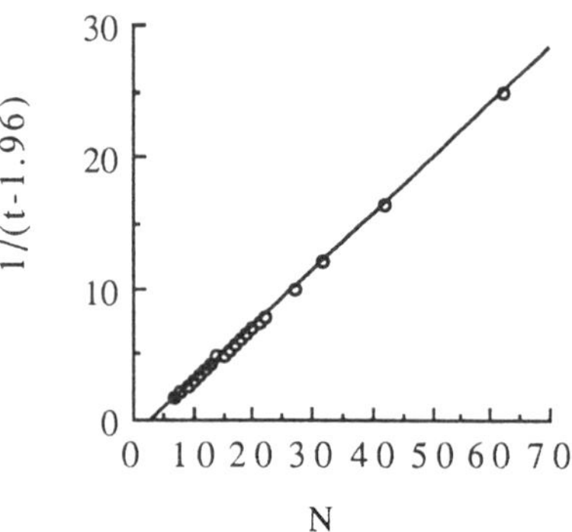

Figure 5.29 Approximation function for *t*.

TABLE 5.24. Program for Testing *t*-Value Approximation.

```
100 FOR N = 7 TO 62 Step 5
110 Y1 = -1.2489 + .42363*N
120 Y2 = 1/Y1
130 Y3 = Y2+1.96
140 PRINT N,Y3
150 NEXT N
```

The calculation has been done via Γ(1.25) since this is an interpolation. It is seen that it corresponds fairly well with the value in the profile and the equation cited above.

(3) It is important to get a "good" fit, since the t-value used in a program should be good to at least three significant figures. t obviously approaches 1.96 as N goes towards infinity, so that the "t-parameter" has to be $t - 1.96$. The graph in Figure 5.29, although one of the transforms is an inverse, is quite good:

$$1/(t - 1.96) = b + aN \tag{5.72}$$

where $b = -1.3489$ and $a = 0.42363$.

The data are checked by the program in BASIC in Table 5.24, and the results in Table 5.25 are obtained.

Aside from the first point, the fit is good. The action recommended would then be to have t-values in the table up to $N = 12$ (df $= 11$) and then use the formula

$$1/(t - 1.96) = -1.3489 + 0.42363*(df + 2) \tag{5.73}$$

or

$$t = 1.96 + \{1/(-1.3489 + 0.42363*(df + 2)\} \tag{5.74}$$

TABLE 5.25. Approximation Function for Student-*t*.

df+2	t(table)	t(approx)
7	2.57	2.54
12	2.228	2.221
17	2.131	2.130
22	2.086	2.084
27	2.060	2.058
32	2.042	2.041
42	2.021	2.020
62	2000	2.000

5.20 REFERENCES

Javaid, K. A. and Cadwallader, D. E., (1972), *J. Pharm. Sci.,* 61:1370.

Lippmann, I., (1972), in *Dissolution Technology,* Eds., Leeson, L. J. and Carstensen, J. T., *The IPT of the Acad. Pharm. Sci.,* Washington, DC, p. 193.

Wagner, J. G., (1969), *J. Pharm. Sci.,* 58:1253.

CHAPTER 6

Normalized Frequency Distributions

THE Gaussian frequency equation was arrived at by curve-fitting means in Chapter 5. In this chapter, the text will concentrate on properties of the Gaussian frequency and distribution functions.

Such terms as standard deviations and means have already been defined. The nomenclature relating to distributions used in this book is as follows: a *frequency function* is one where one states what fraction of a population (or sample) is in a given range. In a batch of a million capsules, the mean may be 100, but some of the capsules may have contents between 98 and 99. It is noted that, when all possible assay or weight values are taken into account and the frequency fractions added up, the sum should be 1.00, i.e., all the capsules.

A *distribution function,* on the other hand, is one where one states the fraction of the population that is smaller than a given value and, in such a case, is denoted an undersize or undersize distribution. Conversely, it could state what fraction is larger than a given value, and then it is an oversize or oversize distribution. Distributions are often said to be (and, indeed, are characterized as being) cumulative.

The modus operandi in investigating distributions and frequency functions commences with a set of samples, and from these samples, one constructs a *histogram.* If data are entered into programs such as StatWorks™ or CricketGraph™, then such histograms can be graphed as bar diagrams.

6.1 HISTOGRAMS

The first question that arises is how many intervals to use. Sturges's rule states that this number is

$$k = 1 + \{3.322 \times \log_{10} [N]\} \tag{6.1}$$

This is then rounded to the nearest (or most convenient) whole number.

TABLE 6.1. Capsule Weights from Random Sampling of a Batch of Capsules.

410, 360, 380, 375, 430, 383, 389, 428, 380, 390, 404, 405,
400, 395, 392, 399, 405, 406, 381, 408, 415, 388, 414, 409
420, 422, 432, 430, 425, 429, 440, 450, 369, 400, 391, 419,
382, 419, 362, 402.

The tabulation then is usually performed by recording the intervals and going through the data, making a mark in the appropriate interval every time a number is encountered. The intervals could be 0–10, 10–20, etc., but the question then arises regarding what to do when the number "10" is arrived at. It is common to interpret this as 0–9.999, 10–19.999, etc. Often, 0–10 is written, with the understanding that 10 belongs in the 10–20 category.

The concept of histograms is best illustrated by the following example.

6.1.1 EXAMPLE 6.1

Given the set of capsule weights in Table 6.1 draw a histogram.

6.1.2 ANSWER 6.1

There are forty pieces of data, so $k = 1 + 3.322 \times \log [40] = 1 + 3.32 \times 1.6 = 1 + 5.3 = 6$. Hence, the set is divided into six categories. The minimum value is 360 and the maximum is 450, so the range is 90; hence, the interval size is 90/6 = 15. The data are tabulated according to this in Table 6.2.

Rather than constructing tables like Table 6.2 from the data as is, it is easier to use a program such as StatWorks™ for arrangement of the data

TABLE 6.2. Data in Table 6.1 Grouped According to Number of Occurrences in the Intervals Given.

Interval	Number of Occurrences
360-375	3
375-390	8
390-405	10
405-420	9
420-435	8
435-450	2

before starting. The data are entered in the order shown in Table 6.1. A suitable heading (e.g., Capsule Weight) is typed in. The column is copied in the second column, and the data file accessed and the address "Rearrange" sought out. The second column is highlighted and okayed, and the column will rearrange in ascending or descending order as requested.

This is then printed, and by using this procedure, the data are presented both in the original and in the systematic order. The arrangement in Table 6.2 is then much easier to make.

6.1.3 EXAMPLE 6.2

Plot histograms of the sets in Table 6.3. Calculate the ordinate value for normal distribution for each interval midpoint.

6.1.4 ANSWER 6.2

Note (and verify) that the number of intervals is correct. Two of the histograms are shown in Figure 6.1. To compare these, it might be worthwhile, first of all, to express the numbers as percent or, even better, as frequencies. This is done in Table 6.4.

Prior to treating this further, it is necessary to discuss the concept of standard deviations a bit further.

6.2 MAKING FREQUENCY DISTRIBUTIONS COMPARABLE

If the data in Table 6.4 are plotted on a common graph (and the end

TABLE 6.3. Three Independent Sets of Data.

Capsule Assays Interval	No	Man Hours Interval	No.	Tablet Weights Interval	No.
<90	0	<200	0	<300	0
90-95	2	200-210	3	300-302	1
95-100	4	210-220	6	302-304	2
100-105	7	220-230	16	304-306	4
105-110	6	230-240	24	306-308	2
110-115	4	240-250	26	308-310	1
115-120	2	250-260	14	>310	0
>120	0	260-270	8		
		270-280	3		
		>280	0		

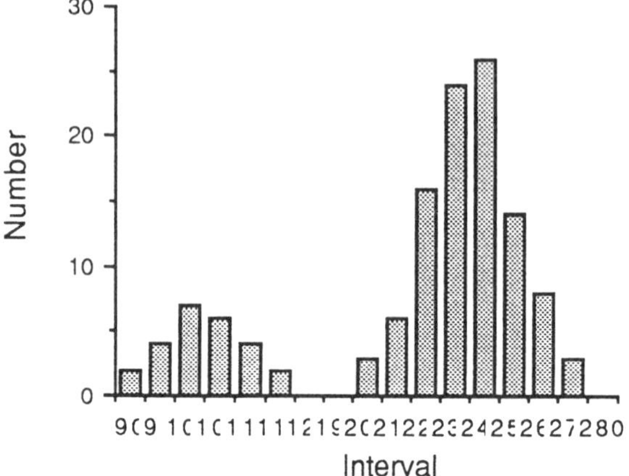

Figure 6.1 Histogram of capsule assays and man hours from Table 6.2.

points of the bars simply connected as a continuous curve), then the graphs would look as shown in Figure 6.2. All these curves are bell-shaped, and the modelistic question that we shall pose is: Is there a common denominator in all of them? Their features are

(1) They are symmetric (about the mean).

(2) The maximum frequency occurs about the mean.

By using an appropriate program (e.g., StatWorks™), the pertinent parameters [mean, standard deviation, and relative standard deviation

TABLE 6.4. Data from Table 6.3 Expressed as Frequencies.

Capsule Assays		Man Hours		Tablet Weights	
Interval	Fraction	Interval	Fraction	Interval	Fraction
<90	0	<200	0	<300	0
90-95	0.08	200-210	0.03	300-302	0.1
95-100	0.16	210-220	0.06	302-304	0.2
100-105	0.28	220-230	0.16	304-306	0.4
105-110	0.24	230-240	0.24	306-308	0.2
110-115	0.08	240-250	0.26	308-310	0.1
115-120	0.08	250-260	0.14	>310	0
>120	0	260-270	0.08		
		270-280	0.03		
		>280	0		

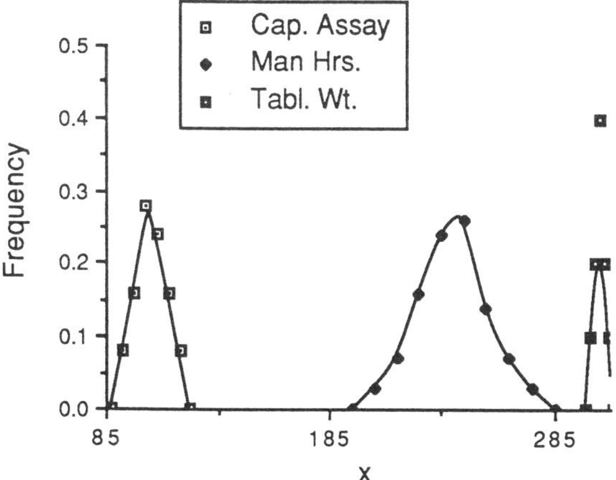

Figure 6.2 Frequency graphs of the data in Table 6.4.

(RSD)] may be calculated, and these are shown in Table 6.5. The data set for man hours is shown in Figure 6.3.

If such plots are constructed for all the data in Table 6.5, it will be noted that a third point about the curves is that

(3) The inflection point is one standard deviation removed from the mean.

To place the curves on a common ground, one could, therefore, make all the midpoints the same by expressing the abscissa (X^*) as a difference from the mean, x_{avg}, i.e.,

$$X^* = x - x_{avg} \tag{6.2}$$

The "spread" of the curves could be equalized by expressing the abscissa (X) in units of standard deviations (by dividing by s), i.e.,

$$Z = (x - x_{avg})/s \tag{6.3}$$

The fact still remains that each of the curves has a different y-value for the peak. The reason for this is that there is a different number of intervals

TABLE 6.5. Means and Standard Deviations of Data in Table 6.4.

Data Set	Mean	Standard Dev.	RSD
Capsule Assay	104.9	6.95	1.59
Man Hours	240.3	15.60	0.52
Tablet Weight	305	2.31	0.38

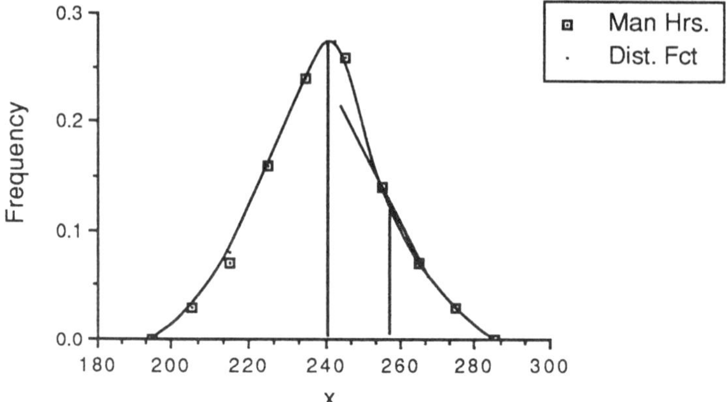

Figure 6.3 Frequency plot of the man-hour figures from Table 6.5.

in each of the original histograms. The way to overcome (or unify) this is to normalize in such a fashion that the areas under the curves are equal. Hence the y-values would be given by the requirement that

$$f = y\Delta X' \qquad \text{or} \qquad y = f/\Delta X' \tag{6.4}$$

where $\Delta X'$ is the interval length. Since in the bar diagram, the values of f add up to 1.000, it follows that the area under the curve will also be 1.000. This treatment of the data in Table 6.4 yields the data in Table 6.6. If y is plotted versus $Z = (x - x_{avg})/s$, then the plot in Figure 6.4 results.

6.3 NORMAL (GAUSSIAN) DISTRIBUTION

The frequency function shown in Figure 6.4 is the normal (Gaussian)

TABLE 6.6. Data from Table 6.4 Normalized.

Capsule Assay			Man Hours			Tablet Weight		
x	(x-x$_{avg}$)/s	y	x	(x-x$_{avg}$)/s	y	x	(x-x$_{avg}$)/s	y
92.5	-1.784	0.111	205	-2.263	0.047	301	-1.732	0.116
97.5	-1.065	0.222	215	-1.622	0.094	303	-0.866	0.231
102.5	-0.345	0.389	225	-0.981	0.250	305	0	0.462
107.5	0.374	0.344	235	-0.340	0.374	307	0.866	0.231
112.5	1.094	0.224	245	0.301	0.406	309	1.731	0.116
117.5	1.813	0.111	255	0.942	0.218			
			265	1.583	0.125			
			275	2.224	0.047			

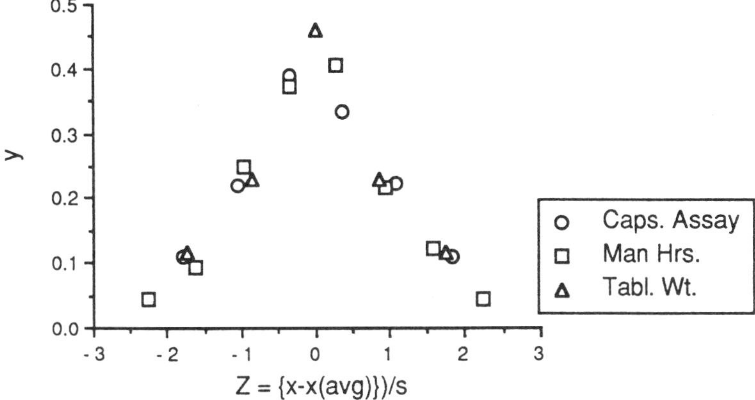

Figure 6.4 The data in Table 6.4 normalized via Equations (6.2) and (6.3).

frequency function with zero mean and unit standard deviation. The equation for this curve is

$$y = (1/(2\pi)^{1/2}) \exp\{(-Z^2/2)\} \qquad (6.5)$$

where Z is defined by Equation (6.2).

This is identical to the equation arrived at in Chapter 5. The curve is normalized, i.e., the area under it is unity, and area values under the curve for different values of Z are to be found in most handbooks. Such a table is shown in Appendix 1. The actual curve is shown in Figure 6.5. If the values of the normal frequency function are desired, then either a table,

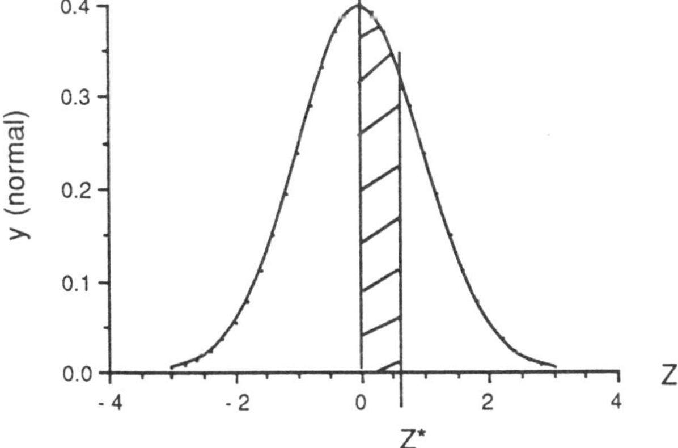

Figure 6.5 The normal (Gaussian) frequency function.

TABLE 6.7. Program for Calculating Ordinate Values of the Gaussian Frequency Function.

```
100  FOR X = -3 TO 3 STEP 0.1
110  Y1  =  1/(2*3.1614)
120  Y2 = Y1*EXP(-(X^2)/2)
130  PRINT X,Y2
140  NEXT X
```

such as shown in Appendix 1, can be consulted, or a simple program for Equation (6.4) can be written. Such a program is shown in Table 6.7. If more values are needed, the value after STEP in step 100 can be changed.

6.4 PROBABILITY CALCULATIONS FROM THE NORMAL DISTRIBUTION

The normal frequency function can be used to calculate probabilities of critical values being reached or superseded. For instance, if the data in Table 6.4 are obtained, various probability calculations can be carried out.

6.4.1 EXAMPLE 6.3

Four sets of data are obtained analytically and accounting-wise and are listed in Table 6.8. The following question may be raised: In set A, what would be the probability of obtaining an assay value above 100.5?

6.4.2 ANSWER 6.3

The normal error table in Appendix 1 is consulted.

"100.5" is 100.5 − 100.23 = 0.27% LC above the mean. The standard deviation is 0.25, so it is 0.27/0.25 = 1.08 standard deviations above the mean.

The *Z*-value corresponds to an area (cross-hatched area in Figure 6.5) of 0.36 or 36%. Since the total area to the right of zero is 50%, the probability of being *above* 1.08 is 50 − 36 = 14%. It is noted that this calculation assumes that the sample under consideration is from a normal population. This is not always true.

6.5 CUMULATIVE PRESENTATION: DISTRIBUTION FUNCTION

The data for capsule assays in Table 6.4 are repeated in Table 6.9 for

TABLE 6.8. Data Set for Analysis.

Set A Initial Assay %L.C.	Set B Drug Content (mg)	Set C Tablet Weight (mg)	Set Man Hours
100.5	20	97.13	18
100.2	55	97.19	20
100.0	48	97.16	15
	52	97.11	22
	51		20
			16
Mean[a]			
100.23	45.2	97.15	18.5
SD[a]			
0.25	14.31	0.035	2.66
Coeff. of Variation[a]			
0.25	31.7	0.026	14.4
SEM[b]			
0.145	6.40	0.0175	1.09

[a]Number of significant figures are exaggerated.
[b]Standard Error of the Mean.

TABLE 6.9. Capsule Assay Data from Table 6.4.

Interval Assay	Frequency	Cumulative Frequency	Percent
<90	0	0	0
90-95	0.08	0.08	8
95-100	0.16	0.24	24
100-105	0.28	0.52	52
105-110	0.24	0.76	76
110-115	0.16	0.92	92
115-120	0.08	1.00	100

convenience. The third column is the cumulative amount less than the lower limit of the interval; for instance, in the 95–100 μm, 16% are less than 100 μm, but the 8% that are less than 95 μm are also less than 100, so that the cumulative amount less than 100 is 8 + 16 = 24%.

When cumulative figures are plotted on probability paper and if the distribution is normal, then a straight line should result. The data are shown as cumulative undersize and cumulative oversize in Figure 6.6. A cumulative curve is, of course, given by the integrated form of the Gaussian equation.

If the data are fairly symmetric, then the difference between plotting oversize or undersize is not great; however, for very scattered data, there can be a difference.

The mean (actually the median) is read off the graph as the point where the line intersects 50%. The standard deviation is obtained as follows.

$Z = 1$ corresponds to an area of 0.3413 (i.e., 68.26% of all measurements is between the mean and plus or minus standard deviation). Hence, reading the abscissa value when the ordinate is 50 − 34 = 16% or 50 + 16 = 86% will give a value that is one standard deviation from the average.

As mentioned, the fourth column is denoted a percent undersize distribution. It is seen in Figure 6.6 that the mean is about 105 and that the standard deviation is about 5. It is also noted that the oversize and undersize distributions give much the same numbers.

6.6 CONSTRUCTION OF PROBABILITY PAPER

Probability paper can be purchased, but any type of purchased paper

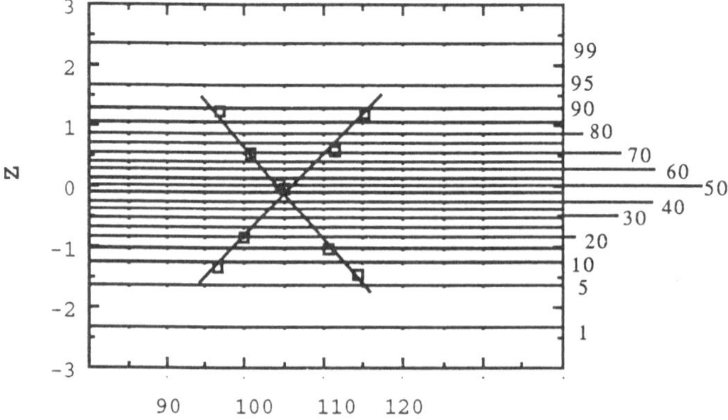

Figure 6.6 Probit presentation of data in Table 6.9.

TABLE 6.10. Data Used for Construction of Probability Paper.

Area	Z-values	Length from the 50% Mark[b]	Ordinate Mark to be Affixed
0	0	0	50%
0.1	0.253	0.433	40% and 60%
0.2	0.534	0.913	30% and 70%
0.3	0.842	1.440	20% and 80%
0.4	1.282	2.192	10% and 90%
0.45	1.645	2.813	5% and 95%
0.49	2.336	3.995	1% and 99%

[a]Values of Z for which the area under the Normal Error Curve is as indicated.
[b]It is assumed that the vertical length of the paper is 8″, so that the half-length is 4″. These 4″ correspond to 2.336 Z-unit, so that one Z-unit is 1.71″.

(other than Cartesian, linear paper) suffers from the fact that one may only use a small section of the paper. Lines on paper should generally have a slope of plus or minus one for presentation purposes so if, for instance, the cumulative figures would all be above 30%, then there would be no need for the "lower" part of the paper. It is therefore useful to know how to construct probability paper.

The normal error table in Appendix 2 is consulted. The Z-values for which the area under the curve is 0.1, 0.2, 0.3, 0.4, 0.45, and 0.49 are sought out. These are listed in Table 6.10. A piece of Cartesian graph paper is used. A 50 is placed in the center of the vertical axis. The values in the last two columns are used to construct the vertical axis.

6.7 PARTICLE SIZES: LOG-NORMAL DISTRIBUTIONS

Most powders (Rodriguez and Carstensen, 1985) are log-normally distributed. Particles, when milled, will usually emerge log-normally distributed (Carstensen and Patel, 1975). Table 6.11 and Figure 6.7 are examples of this.

The mean diameter, d_g, called the geometric mean diameter, is given by

$$\ln [d_g] = (1/N)\Sigma N_i \ln [d_i] \tag{6.6}$$

or

$$[d_g] = \Pi[d_i]^{Ni/N} \tag{6.7}$$

TABLE 6.11. Particle Size Distribution of Griseofulvin.

Diameter (μm), d	Percent Above by Number	ln[d]
2	99	0.693
6	90	1.792
10	70	2.303
18	50	2.890
25	30	3.219
35	20	3.555
55	10	4.007

where Π stands for multiplicative "summation." It is by way of Equation (6.6) that the term "geometric" or "harmonic" mean is used for this parameter.

To get the standard deviation, just as in the case of normal distributions, one reads off the value at $Z = -1$ or at 16%, and the number obtained is a logarithmic number. This value is the same whether one uses 16% or 84%. However, if the antilogarithm is taken, the number differs. It is therefore commonplace to denote the standard deviation of a log-normal distribution by ln [s].

6.7.1 EXAMPLE 6.4

Determine the values of the geometric mean diameter, the standard devi-

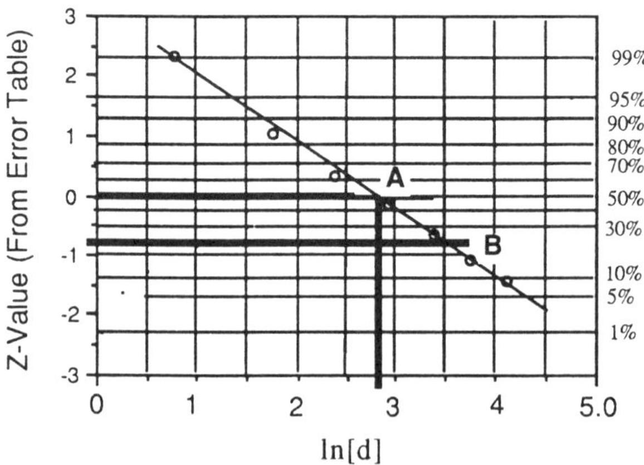

Figure 6.7 Data from Table 6.7 plotted on probability paper using logarithmic scale. The right ordinate indicates percent oversize.

ation, and the values of the diameter at the mean plus or minus one standard deviation in Figure 6.7.

6.7.2 ANSWER 6.4

The logarithm of the mean diameter is read off the graph to be

$$\ln [d_g] = 2.8, \qquad \text{so} \qquad d_g = \exp(2.8) = 16.4$$

$Z = 1$ (16%) occurs at point B or $\ln [d] = 3.6$, so

$$\ln [s] = 3.6 - 2.8 = 0.8$$

At minus one standard deviation, therefore,

$$d_{-s} = \exp(2.8 - 0.8) = 7.4$$

and at plus one standard deviation

$$d_{+s} = \exp(3.6) = 36.6$$

It is noted that 16.4 is not the midpoint between 36.6 and 7.4.

6.8 STATISTICAL MOMENTS

Using the notation t for the standard normal deviate, it has been seen above that the Gaussian frequency function is normalized to unit area, i.e.,

$$F(0) = (1/(2\pi)^{1/2}) \int_{-\infty}^{\infty} \exp\{(-t^2/2)\} = 1 \qquad (6.8)$$

The distribution, as mentioned, is symmetrical. Many programs (such as StatWorks™) give information not only about this, but also about the skewness and the kurtosis of a set of data presented to it. These properties are associated with the so-called moments of a function. The moments are defined as

$$M_x(\phi) = \text{ave}[e^{\phi x}] = \int_{-\infty}^{\infty} e^{\phi x} f(x) dx \qquad (6.9)$$

where $f(x)$ is the frequency function. The first moment is μ, and the mean of the population and the second moment is σ^2, the variance of the population. The third moment is related to the semi-invariant k_3 given by

$$k_3 = \{n^2S_3 - 3nS_2S_1 + 2S_1^2\}/\{\sigma^2[n(n - 1)(n - 2)]\} \quad (6.10)$$

and is often used as a measure of skewness.

The use of moments in pharmaceutical applications is rare. Carstensen et al. (1970) have used the principle to show that, when a drug is added to (dusted into) a sugar coat, then the content uniformity will be better if many (N) small applications are used than if a few (n) large applications are made. The variances will be proportional to N/n.

6.9 REFERENCES

Carstensen, J. T., Koff, A., Johnson, J. and Rubin, S., (1970), *J. Pharm, Sci.*, 59:553.
Carstensen, J. T. and Patel, M. R., (1975), *J. Pharm. Sci.*, 64:1494.
Rodriguez, N. and Carstensen, J. T., (1985), *J. Pharm. Sci.*, 74:1322.

CHAPTER 7

Other Distributions

IT has been seen that there are other distributions than the normal, e.g., log-normal distributions and F-distributions. The chapter to follow deals with a series of fairly important distributions.

7.1 POPULATIONS

So far, we have dealt with samples. As an example, it is assumed that a batch is made of twenty capsules with the drug contents shown in Table 7.1.

This is a *population,* i.e., all possible numbers are included in it. The number of degrees of freedom of this is N (since no estimates have to be calculated), and the *population variance,* denoted σ^2, is given by

$$\sigma^2 = SS/N \tag{7.1}$$

and a similar expression for the *population standard deviation:*

$$\sigma = [SS/N]^{1/2} \tag{7.2}$$

The population mean is denoted μ and is the average of the above figures. In the above example,

$$\mu = 96.8 \tag{7.3}$$

$$\sigma^2 = 23.67 \tag{7.4}$$

$$\sigma = 4.865 \tag{7.5}$$

When using calculators or programs, it is always important to check

TABLE 7.1. Ten Capsules Constituting a Population.

Capsule	Content	Capsule	Content
A	90	K	95
B	90	L	95
C	90	M	102
D	90	N	102
E	95	O	102
F	95	P	102
G	95	Q	102
H	95	R	102
I	95	S	102
J	95	T	102

whether the number for "standard deviation" denotes σ (divisor N) or s (divisor $N - 1$).

We rarely, if ever, know the totality of the population. Most tests are destructive (e.g., a chemical assay), and hence, the only manner in which the entire population (e.g., of 1,000,000 capsules) could be determined would be to assay them all.

For this reason, it is necessary to take a *sample*. It is assumed that the sample mean and standard deviation are best estimators (denoted $E\{\ \}$) of the population mean and standard deviation, i.e.,

$$s = E\{\sigma\} \tag{7.6}$$

$$x_{\text{avg}} = E\{\mu\} \tag{7.7}$$

They, of course, will rarely be the same as the population parameters, and we would like to state with a certain level of confidence how close they may be to the population parameters. This is associated with calculations that lead to statements such as: The population standard deviation is in the interval $S \pm Q$, where Q is a calculated figure such that the statement has a certain probability of being correct.

Conventionally, Q is calculated such that it represents 95% confidence; i.e., in making a similar calculation and statement twenty times, one will be wrong, on the average, once. Whenever making such statements, these words should be placed in a footnote, to cover the authors in the one case of twenty when she/he is wrong. It is a lemma of Murphy's law that one is always remembered for the few times one is wrong, not the many times one is right.

Suppose that the capsules in Table 7.1 are at hand, and it is desired to sample them to ascertain what the content is (by chemical assay), and let us assume that the assay method is completely accurate and precise. If samples of three are taken, then the combinations shown in Table 7.2 are possible. It is seen, hence, that the standard deviation can take on five distinct numbers (0, 2.89, 6.93, 6.02, and 4.04). It should be noted that these would not occur with equal probability. For instance, the probability of 90, 90, 90 is considerably smaller than the probability of the other constellations. There is quite a spread in the standard deviations, and it is obvious that if the sample at hand is the only source of information regarding the standard deviation, then this latter is not a very precise number.

7.2 THE χ^2-DISTRIBUTION, CONFIDENCE INTERVALS

To estimate how precise the standard deviation is, it is necessary to know how standard deviations are distributed. The distribution in question is actually the distribution of the sums of squares from which the standard deviation is calculated.

This is the so-called χ^2-distribution and normalized sums of squares, in general, are distributed by this distribution. A normalized sum of squares is the SS ($= (n - 1)s^2$) divided by the population variance (σ^2). To obtain the 95% confidence limits, a table for the 0.025 and the 0.975 value of χ^2 is consulted for the particular degrees of freedom. A table of χ^2-values for various degrees of freedom is shown in Appendix 8.

TABLE 7.2. Possible Combinations of the Data in Table 6.1 When Sampled in a Size of Three.

Combination			Mean	St.Dev.
90	90	90	90	0
90	90	95	92.67	2.89
90	95	95	98.33	2.89
90	90	102	94	6.93
90	102	102	98	6.93
90	95	102	95.67	6.02
95	95	95	95	0
95	95	102	97.33	4.04
95	102	102	99.67	4.04
102	102	102	102	0

In the above case $n - 1 = 2$, and the values for χ^2 are

$$\chi^2_{0.025} = 0.0506 \tag{7.8}$$

$$\chi^2_{0.975} = 7.378 \tag{7.9}$$

Since the normalized sum of squares is between these two numbers one may write:

$$\chi^2_{0.025} < (n - 1)s^2/\sigma^2 < \chi^2_{0.975} \tag{7.10}$$

or

$$s^2(n - 1)/\chi^2_{0.025} > \sigma^2 > s^2(n - 1)/\chi^2_{0.975} \tag{7.11}$$

Taking, for instance, the fifth set (90, 95, 100), the standard deviation is 5.0; i.e., the variance is 25 and the sum of squares is 50. Hence, Equation (7.11) will read

$$50/0.0506 = 988 > \sigma^2 > 50/7.378 = 6.77 \tag{7.12}$$

or

$$31 > \sigma > 2.6 \tag{7.13}$$

This is obviously a rather large interval. It may (on the surface) seem odd that it does not include zero (which is one of the occurrences in Table 7.2, albeit at low probability). But it should be emphasized that it is the population standard deviation that is in the interval in Equation (7.13) An exception is the case where zero standard deviation is noted. $s = 0$ is an artifact of the numbers (which are constructed), and a zero standard deviation in real life is quite unlikely.

The wide interval in Equation (7.13) shows that if the sample at hand is the only source for an estimate of the population variance, then the number will be rather imprecise.

If a larger sample were taken, then the situation would be more precise, e.g., for a set of eight,

$$90,\ 90,\ 95,\ 95,\ 95,\ 95,\ 102,\ 102 \tag{7.14}$$

the variance is 20.86, so that the sum of squares is $7 \times 20.86 = 146$. The χ^2-values (with 7 df) are 16.03 and 1.69, so that the interval in which the population variance lies is calculated to be

$$146/1.69 = 146 > \sigma^2 > 146/16.03 = 9.1 \tag{7.15}$$

or

$$12 > \sigma > 3 \tag{7.16}$$

If the sample at hand, therefore, is the only source of a standard deviation, then the interval in Equation (7.16) will be wide. Even with a larger sample, say with degrees of freedom of 20, the χ^2-values would be 9.951 and 34.17, and in this case a sum of squares of 146 would have given an interval of $10 > \sigma > 2$. If, for instance, an assay has been carried out often and a pooled standard deviation with many degrees of freedom is available, then the interval will be more reasonable.

7.3 OUTLIERS

An excellent procedure for testing for outliers is the one of Natrella (1963). Consider, for instance, the following set of numbers:

$$20, 55, 48, 52, 51 \tag{7.17}$$

One might wonder if there is something "wrong" with the value 20 and if it would be permissible to discard it. There are methods for this, and they depend on whether the sample at hand is the only source of information regarding the standard deviation or whether there are other data that can be used to estimate the standard deviation.

Suppose the sample in Equation (7.17) is the only time the test has been carried out. This could be a sample tested in preformulation (where not much material is at hand), or it could be a sample used in a screening study to see if a certain variable in a system was significant. In such a case, the so-called Dixon procedure is used:

(1) One first arranges the values in ascending order, denoting the smallest number A_1 and the largest number A_n.
(2) One then chooses the probability one is willing to take of ejecting a number that actually belongs in the group. This is usually set at 5%.
(3) One then calculates a number, r_{ij}, as shown in Table 7.3.
(4) r_{ij} is calculated in the manner shown in Table 7.4.
(5) One now seeks the value of r_{ij} for the appropriate $r_{1-\alpha}$ value in the table in Appendix 6. If $r_{ij} > r_{1-\alpha}$, then the suspect value can be rejected.

TABLE 7.3. Table for Outliers.

Sample Size	r_{ij} Applicable	Equation
$3 \leq n \leq 7$	Calculate r_{10}	(7.22)
$8 \leq n \leq 10$	Calculate r_{11}	(7.23)
$11 \leq n \leq 13$	Calculate r_{21}	(7.24)
$14 \leq n \leq 23$	Calculate r_{22}	(7.25)

In the example in Equation (7.17), the numbers are placed in ascending order:

$$20,\ 48,\ 52,\ 51,\ 55 \tag{7.18}$$

and, since the lowest number is suspect, it follows that

$$r_{10} = (48 - 20)/(55 - 20) = 0.8 > r_{ij}(\text{crit}) = 0.765 \tag{7.19}$$

where the critical value has been obtained from Appendix 6 at 4 df and 95% upper percentile. The value 20 may be rejected.

7.3.1 EXAMPLE 7.1

If the lowest value had been 30 and not 20, could it have been rejected at the 95% confidence level?

7.3.2 ANSWER 7.1

$$r_{10} = (48 - 30)/(55 - 30) = 0.72 < r_{ij}(\text{crit}) = 0.642 \tag{7.20}$$

so that this value could not have been rejected.

It is noted that the largest (small) value that can be rejected is given by

$$(48 - x)/(55 - x) = 0.765 \tag{7.21}$$

TABLE 7.4. Formulae for Calculating r_{ij}.

r_{ij}	Only Largest Number (A_n) Suspect	Only Smallest Number (A_1) Suspect	Eq. No
r_{10}	$(A_n-A_{n-1})/(A_n-A_1)$	$(A_2-A_1)/(A_n-A_1)$	(7.26)
r_{11}	$(A_n-A_{n-1})/(A_n-A_2)$	$(A_2-A_1)/(A_{n-1}-A_1)$	(7.27)
r_{21}	$(A_n-A_{n-2})/(A_n-A_2)$	$(A_2-A_1)/(A_{n-1}-A_1)$	(7.28)
r_{22}	$(A_n-A_{n-2})/(A_n-A_2)$	$(A_2-A_1)/(A_{n-2}-A_1)$	(7.29)

or

$$X = 25.5 \tag{7.22}$$

If there is another source of information regarding the standard deviation, then a different procedure is used, and the critical values for this are listed in Appendix 7.

Suppose a graduate scientist has performed an assay of the above type three times five times (i.e., replicates of five) and found the pooled standard deviation to be 2.96 with 12 df.

In this case, one proceeds with steps (1) and (2) above and then

(3) The value of $q_{1-\alpha}\ (n,\nu)$ is looked up in Appendix 7, where n is the number of observations in the sample (i.e., in this case 5) and where ν is the df for s, the independent estimate of the standard deviation (i.e., in this case 12).

(4) The value of $Q = q_{1-\alpha}s$ is then calculated.

(5) If $A_n - A_1 > Q$, then the value is discarded.

In the case in Equation (7.17) with the stipulations in the preceding paragraph, the value of $q_{1-\alpha}$ is found for 95% and df = 12 to be 4.51, so

$$Q = 4.51 \times 2.96 = 13.3 \tag{7.23}$$

Since

$$A_n - A_1 = 35 > 13.3 \tag{7.24}$$

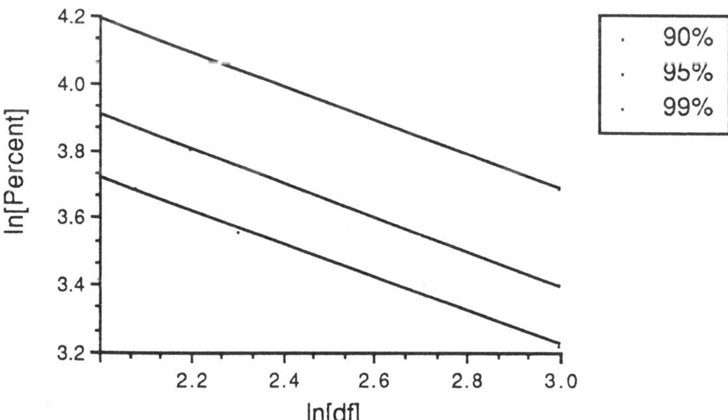

Figure 7.1 The df needed to obtain the sd within a certain percentage of its true value with a given degree of confidence. Constructed from data published by Greenwood and Sandomire (1950).

to truncate the 95% confidence interval at one (at most, two) significant figures, and this then implies the significant figures in the average as well.

7.6.3 EXAMPLE 7.3

Given the second set of data in Table 7.5 (set C2), state the average and the 95% confidence interval.

7.6.4 ANSWER 7.3

In a manner similar to previously, the interval is found to be 3.21, so that the 95% confidence limits are

$$51.2 \pm 3.21 \tag{7.28}$$

But the value 3.21 should be given with only one significant figure; therefore, the average (51.2) cannot be given with more significant figures, so that the correct way of stating the interval is

$$51 \pm 3 \tag{7.29}$$

It is an old-fashioned custom to imply one more number but made as a subscript, i.e., state

$$51._2 \pm 3._2 \tag{7.30}$$

Nowadays, scientists are rather careless with significant numbers, and as a general rule, people, without assessment, use three significant figures without being reproached by their peers. In certain instances (weights, for instance), many more figures are significant. But to be careless and give more than three figures if it is not justified may cause adverse comment and reflect on the credibility of the published work containing the data.

7.7 THE BINOMIAL DISTRIBUTION

If a batch of well-blended powder was sampled to test whether the content were indeed what was claimed, then, since the sample is particulate (heterogeneous), there will be an uncertainty related to the size of the sample. If, in the ridiculous extreme, it is decided to take a sample of three particles from a blend containing 40% ($p = 0.4$) of active drug, then the probability of obtaining a sample containing zero drug particles would be 0.6^3, i.e., finite.

Given a population with a fraction, p, of drug (probability of success), if a sample of size N (N particles, N tries) is taken, then the probability of picking a sample with x drug particles (successes) is

$$\Pr(x) = \left[{N \atop x}\right] p^x(1 - p)^{N-x} \tag{7.31}$$

where $\left[{N \atop x}\right]$ is the number of ways in which x articles can be removed from N articles. It is given by the binomial formula

$$\left[{N \atop x}\right] = N!/((N - x)!x!) \tag{7.32}$$

The average number is

$$\text{avg}(x) = Np \tag{7.33}$$

and the variance is

$$\text{var}(x) = p(1 - p)/N \tag{7.34}$$

7.7.1 EXAMPLE 7.4

A batch of powder contains 0.3 = 30% of drug. Samples of three are taken. What are the possible outcomes, and what are their probabilities?

7.7.2 ANSWER 7.4

The binomial probabilities for $p = 0.3$ and $N - 3$ are shown in Table 7.6.

TABLE 7.6. Binomial Probabilities for $p = 0.3$ and $N = 3$.

No of Drug Particles	$p^x(1-p)^{N-x}$.	$[N_x]$	Probability
0	0.343	1	0.343
1	0.147	3	0.441
2	0.063	3	0.189
3	0.027	1	0.027
Total			1.000

7.8 PROBLEM

(1) A specialty product consists of very small tablets, 30% of which are placebo and 70% of which are active. The small tablets are mixed and placed in a hopper (complete homogeneity assumed). They are then filled into capsules. Assume that this is a random action, and calculate the probabilities of getting 0, 1, 2,. . . , N active tablets in the capsule, for

- $N = 4$
- $N = 5$
- $N = 6$
- $N = 7$
- $N = 8$

Plot these on probability paper and

(1) Comment on the linearity.

(2) Compare the mean and the theoretical mean.

(3) Compare the sd with the theoretical (binomial) sd.

7.9 ANSWER

(1) The probabilities for $N = 8$ are listed in Table 7.7 with the appropriate binomial coefficients. The expression for the probability of picking x from N, when the fraction of X is p, is $\Pr(x) = [N_x]p^x(1-p)^{N-x}$ is

$$\text{avg}\ (x) = Np = 8x = 0.24$$

TABLE 7.7. Probabilities for $N = 8$ and $p = 0.3$ in a Binomial Distribution.

q	$p^x(1-p)^{8-x}$.	[8 x]	Probability	Cumulative >
8	0.0000656	1	0.0000656	0.999881
7	0.0001531	8	0.0012312	0.998750
6	0.0003572	28	0.0100019	0.988748
5	0.0008335	56	0.046676	0.942072
4	0.0019448	70	0.1361367	0.805936
3	0.00453789	56	0.2541218	0.551814
2	0.01058841	28	0.2964755	0.255339
1	0.02470629	8	0.1976503	0.057688
0	0.057648	1	0.0576880	
Total				1.000047

and the standard deviation is

$$\text{var}(x) = p(1 - p)/N = 0.3 \times 0.7 \times 8 = 1.6$$

Both of these figures are in good agreement with the data if the last column is plotted cumulatively on probability paper.

7.10 REFERENCES

Gosset, P., (1908), *Biometrika,* VI:1–25.

Greenwood, J. A. and Sandomire, M. M., (1950), *J. Am. Stat. Assoc.,* 5:258.

Natrella, M., (1963), *Experimental Statistics,* U.S. Dept. of Commerce, NBS, pp. 17-1–17-6.

CHAPTER 8

Significance Testing

IT has been shown in previous chapters that "differences" are often the substance of scientific probing. The question is, then, if two experiments give different values (and the values will always be "somewhat" different), is this difference meaningful? The distributions described in the previous chapter can be used to determine whether two events, sets of data, averages, dispersions, etc., are significantly different or not.

At the onset, let it be said that the principle used (the Null hypothesis) is such that, by performing a certain set of tests, one will either

(1) Show a significant difference on a given confidence level
(2) Or fail to show such a difference

It is to be noted that

(3) One never shows that two events or numbers are equal.[12]
(4) If one fails to show a difference with one test, but shows a significant difference with another test, then there is (at the given level of confidence) a significant difference.

8.1 NULL HYPOTHESIS

In the task of comparing numbers, one starts out with the hypothesis that the two numbers are the same. (The difference is null; i.e., if the means are being compared, it is assumed at the onset that $\mu_1 = \mu_2$.) This is expressed as

$$H_0: \qquad \mu_1 = \mu_2 \tag{8.1}$$

[12]At best, one shows equivalence, which essentially is failure to show a significant difference at a certain confidence level.

Calculations of the probability of this being correct are then carried out, and if the probability (α) is small, then one accepts the alternate hypothesis:

$$H_a: \quad \mu_1 \neq \mu_2 \tag{8.2}$$

α is the probability of being correct with the null hypotheses and wrong with the alternate hypotheses. α is usually (and in this text, in general) set at 0.05 or 5%.

8.2 TESTING BY COMPARING VARIANCES

One manner in which one might probe this is to ask what the sample standard deviation is, and to this end, one would, in general, calculate the pooled standard deviation. As mentioned at an earlier point, the standard deviation of the average, the so-called standard error of the mean (sem) is given by the sample standard deviation (s) divided by the square root of the number of determinations in the set (N), i.e.,

$$\text{sem} = s/\sqrt{N} \tag{8.3}$$

Similarly, the variance of the average would be

$$\text{sem}^2 = s^2/N \tag{8.4}$$

If, for example, one had three sets of triplicate measurements, as shown in Table 8.1, one might calculate both the pooled standard deviation and then calculate the standard deviation of the averages. The two should correlate in the manner of Equation (8.3).

If a variance is obtained in two different manners, then the ratio of the variances is distributed by an F-distribution, with the respective degrees of

TABLE 8.1. Rate Constants at Three Different Levels of Salt Concentration.

	Set A	Set B	Set C
	0.12	0.11	0.17
	0.14	0.13	0.13
	0.11	0.15	0.14
Avg	0.1233	0.13	0.1467
s^2	0.00063	0.00040	0.000433

freedom. In the above example, the pooled sample variance is found to be

$$s^2_{\text{pooled}} = 0.000354 \text{ (with 6 df)} \tag{8.5}$$

or an estimate of sem² of

$$E(\text{sem}^2) = 0.000354/3 = 0.000118 \tag{8.6}$$

and the averages have a mean of 0.13 and a variance of

$$s^2_{\text{avg}} = 0.000279 \text{ (with 2 df)} \tag{8.7}$$

The question then is: Are these really different? The scientist carrying out the experiment may have a "feeling" that there is a trend in the data, since the rate constant increases with salt concentration (kinetic ionic strength effect), but can he really claim this?

In forming the ratio of the variances, it is customary to place the larger number in the numerator, and we find that

$$s^2_{\text{avg}}/s^2_{\text{pooled}} = 2.36 \tag{8.8}$$

Consulting the *F*-table (95% confidence) in Appendix 5, we find that

$$F_{\text{crit}} \text{ (2 df,6 df)} = 5.14 > 2.36 \tag{8.9}$$

so that it is not justifiable, by this test, to state that the values are "different" on the 95% confidence level.

The example above was simple in the sense that each set had the same number of determinations. In the common case, the sets A, B, and C may not have the same number of determinations, and this complicates matters.

8.3 THE *F*-TEST

In the *F*-test, the pooled standard deviation is calculated and is usually denoted s_w ("w" standing for within). The value corresponding to sem² in the above is denoted s_b^2 ("b" for between) and is given by

$$s_b^2 = \{1/(K - 1)\}\{(T_1^2/N_1) + (T_2^2/N_2) + \ldots - (\Sigma T_i^2/\Sigma N_i)\} \tag{8.10}$$

where T_i denotes the sum of the values in the *i*th column and N_i denotes the number of data in the *i*th column. *K* is the number of sets. An example will illustrate this: Given the assays of three batches, A, B, and C in Table 8.2, it is desired to determine whether there is a significant difference between them.

$$s_w^2 = (0.2 + 0.3 + 0.475)/(3 + 4 + 5)$$

$$= 0.975/12 = 0.08125 \text{ (df} = 12)$$

$$s_b^2 = \{1/(3 - 1)\}[2500 + 3001.25 + 3947.535$$

$$- 9445.130\underline{6}] = 3.654334$$

It is to be noted that the term in the square brackets constitutes a small difference between large numbers, so it is necessary to carry many places after the decimal. Hence, the variance ratio is VR = $s_w^2/s_w^2 = 45 > 3.89 = F_{crit}(2,12)$ so that a significant difference within the sets is established on the 95% level.

8.4 FACTORIALS

Frequently, it is important to assess whether a variable in a study is "of

TABLE 8.2. Assays of Three Batches, A, B, and C.

	Set A	Set B	Set C
	25.1	24.5	25.7
	24.9	24.6	25.4
	24.7	24.2	25.9
	25.3	24.9	25.5
		24.3	25.3
			26.1
Avg	25	24.5	25.65
Total	100	122.5	153.9
T^2/N	2500	3001.25	3947.535
Grand Total, GT			376.4
$(GT)^2/N$			9445.1307
Variance	0.0$\underline{6}$.	0.075	0.095
SS	0.2	0.3	0.475
n - 1	3	4	5

TABLE 8.3. Effect of Compression Pressure and of Lubricant Level on Disintegration Time (min) of a Tablet Product.

	High Pressure	Low Pressure	Totals
With Lubricant	71 and 69	51 and 49	240
Without Lubricant	71 and 69	51 and 49	240
Totals	280	200	480

importance" or not. In such a case, it is customary, if the number of variables is not excessive, to carry out the experiment at two (or, at times, three) levels. If there are N variables and each is carried out at two levels, then the number of experiments in the "full" factorial is N^2. For five variables, for instance, sixty-four measurements would be necessary.

An example is shown of a 2^2 factorial in Table 8.3, where the variables in a tablet experiment are lubricant and compression pressure and where the "response" (i.e., the quality investigated) is the disintegration of the produced tablets. Each measurement is carried out in duplicate as shown. In this case, the lubricant makes no difference. Hence, the value for s_w could be obtained from the two sets:

71,69,61,69 and 51,49,51,49

with df = 3 + 3 = 6.

There is an effect of the pressure, which, when estimated, consumes one degree of freedom. The total number of degrees of freedom is 8 − 1 = 7, so an accounting of the degrees of freedom assigned to the effects is shown in Table 8.4. Note that the degrees of freedom of the error has been obtained from the total minus that of the effect (and hence is parenthesized).

Usually, a disintegrant is added to tablet formulations, and a situation, different from the one in Table 8.3 is shown in Table 8.5 where there *is* an effect of magnesium stearate. The possible effects are as follows:

- starch: 121 + 37 = 158 versus 119 + 43 = 162
- pressure: 200 versus 120
- lubricant: 121 + 119 = 240 versus 37 + 43 = 80

TABLE 8.4. Summary of Data in Table 8.3.

Effect	Degrees of Freedom
Pressure	1
Residual	(6)
Total	7

TABLE 8.5. Effect of Compression Pressure and of Lubricant Level on Disintegration Time (min) of a Tablet Product.

	High Pressure	Low Pressure	Totals
With Lubricant +St	71	50	121
Lubricant No Starch	69	50	119
Total With Lubricant			240
No Lubricant + St	29	8	37
No Lub No Starch	31	12	43
Total, No Lubricant			80
Totals	200	120	320

The degrees of freedom are assigned as shown in Table 8.6. The method to follow is denoted Analysis of Variance (ANOVA).

The question, then, is whether these effects are significant. To this end, their mean sum of squares, MS (sum of squares divided by degrees of freedom), are calculated. It is noted that two levels are involved in all of the above, so each of the effects has $2 - 1 = 1$ df.

The sum of squares for the three effects (pressure: SS_P; lubricant: SS_L; and starch: SS_S) are

$$SS_S = (158^2/4) + (162^2/4) - (320^2/4)$$

$$= 6{,}241 + 6{,}561 - 12{,}800 = 2$$

$$SS_L = (240^2/4) + (80^2/4) - (320^2/8)$$

$$= 14{,}400 + 1{,}600 - 12{,}800 = 3{,}200$$

$$SS_P = (200^2/4) + (120^2/4) - (320^2/8)$$

$$= 10{,}000 + 3{,}600 - 12{,}800 = 800$$

TABLE 8.6. Degrees of Freedom Assigned.

Effect	Degrees of Freedom
Pressure	1
Mag. Stearate	1
Cornstarch	1
Residual	(4)
Total	7

TABLE 8.7. ANOVA Table for Three Effects.

Effect	SS	df	MS	VR	$F_{crit.}$
Starch	2	1	2	6.66	6.61
Lubricant	800	1	800	533	6.61
Pressure	3,200	1	3,200	4,267	6.61
Residual	6	(8)	(0.75)		
Total	4,008	7			

The total sum of squares (7 × the variance of the numbers taken individually) is 4.008, and the ANOVA table then becomes like that shown in Table 8.7. The numbers in parentheses have been obtained by difference. Hence, for the degrees of freedom, the total is $N - 1$, when there are a total of N numbers in the whole box. One is assigned to each effect, and the degree of freedom assigned to the residual is the difference.

One next calculates the sums of squares for each of the effects and for the residual by taking the sum of squares and subtracting the grand total squared divided by N. This divided by df is the MS, which is then divided by that of the residual, to give a variance ratio (VR), which is compared with that of F_{crit} for the appropriate degrees of freedom.

It is seen that the effect of the starch is barely (and probably not) significant. The two other effects are significant on a high level of significance. Assuming that the starch has no effect and that the only two effects are that of pressure and that of lubricant, a new ANOVA table can be constructed (and, at times, effects that were marginal become significant).

8.5 DIFFERENCES BETWEEN ESTIMATES OF s

If an experiment is repeated, then the standard deviation will (most often) be different from what it was the first time around. The question is whether the second standard deviation was really different or whether it was simply a question of experimental error that gave rise to the two different numbers. To test whether there is a significant difference between two standard deviations, the ratio of the variances is determined. The ratio is distributed by an F-distribution. Values for the F-distribution are shown in Appendix 5.

8.5.1 EXAMPLE 8.1

Given the sets of numbers in Table 8.8, determine whether there is a significant difference between the standard deviations.

TABLE 8.8. Assay Figures from a Pharmaceutical Product.

	Assay A	Assay B	Assay C	Assay D
	15.2	14.2	13.2	13.2
	15.0	14.9	13.0	13.0
	15.8	14.9	13.8	13.8
	14.2	15.0	14.2	14.2
		14.5		14.5
		14.8		14.7
s^2	0.436	0.094	0.303	0.480
N-1	3	5	3	5
SS	1.31	0.47	0.91	2.1

8.5.2 ANSWER 8.1

The worst ratio is

$$R = 0.48/0.094 = 4.9 < F_{crit,0.95}(5,5) = 5.05$$

Hence, it is not justified to state that there is a significant difference between the two variances.

8.6 THE UNPAIRED *t*-TEST: SAMPLES AT HAND THE ONLY SOURCE OF VARIANCE

The *t*-test for estimating whether there are "differences" between acquired numbers is probably the most common significance test used. As an example, four sets of numbers (assay per tablet of several clinical batches), A–F, are shown in Table 8.9.

TABLE 8.9. Assay Figures from a Pharmaceutical Product.

	Set A	Set B	Set C	Set D	Set E	Set F
1	10.50	11.00	13.6	12.5	10.50	13.1
2.	10.45	11.90	12.9	12.6	10.45	12.7
3.	10.10	11.20	12.5	12.5	10.10	11.6
4.	10.00	11.25	13.5	12.4	10.00	12.6
5.	10.10	11.00	14.0	12.5		12.3
Avg.	10.23	11.27	13.33	12.5	10.26	12.46
Var.	0.052	0.137	0.355	0.05	0.062	0.313
sem	0.102	0.166	0.266	0.0317	0.125	0.250
sd	0.228	0.370	0.396	0.071	0.25	0.559

Considering sets B and E, one might ask: Are the sets different? Are the means different? This can be answered by carrying out a *t*-test. In this, there are the following steps for the means (X_1 and X_2) of two sets with *m* and *n* data points:

(1) One ascertains (by forming the ratio of variances and comparing them to the appropriate value of *F*) that there are no significant differences between the variances of the two sets. If there were, then one would automatically have shown that the two sets did not come from the same population, although the data might not suffice to show that the averages were different.

(2) If the *F*-test fails to show a significant difference between the means on the 95% confidence level, then one proceeds to test whether there is a significant difference between the means in the following manner.

(3) One decides the level of confidence on which one wishes to express one's decision (i.e., are the means different?). This is usually 95% or $\alpha = 0.05$.

(4) One computes the pooled standard deviation, s_w (which has $\nu = n + m - 2$ df). For two sets with *m* and *n* determinations, one may now write

$$s_w^2 = (s_1^2 n_1 + s_2^2 m_2)/(n + m - 2) \qquad (8.11)$$

(5) One computes the following parameter (Youden, 1951):

$$t = \{(X_1 - X_2)/s\}[nm/(n + m)]^{1/2} \qquad (8.12)$$

(6) The differences between the averages have this student *t*-value, and if the difference $\pm t$ includes zero, then one may not state that it is different from zero. Hence, if *t* is larger than the two-sided $t_{1-\alpha,\nu}$-value, then there is a significant difference between the two sets on the $100(1 - (\alpha/2))\%$ confidence level.

8.6.1 EXAMPLE 8.2

Is there a significant difference on the 95% confidence level between sets B and E?

8.6.2 ANSWER 8.2

The ratio between the variances is $0.137/0.062 = 2.22 < F_{0.95,3,4} = 9.12$.

The pooled variance is $[(4 \times 0.062) + (5 \times 0.137)]/(3 + 4) = 0.134$; i.e., the pooled sd is

$$s = 0.37 \tag{8.13}$$

$$t = \{(11.27 - 10.26)/0.37\} \times [(4 \times 5)/9]^{1/2} = 4.06 \tag{8.14}$$

This is larger than the t for 7 df on the 99% level (not shown in tables here). By use of StatWorks™, the output in Table 8.10 is obtained by the following procedure: The two sets of data to be compared are entered in the table that appears when the program is called up. The File "STAT" is moused out, and the mouse is dragged to the file addressed "t-Test." The various entry headings (set A, set B, etc.) will appear in two columns. The two sets to be compared are highlighted, one in one column, the other in the other. One opts between "paired" or "nonpaired" by highlighting the choice circles. The OK is then highlighted, and a printout such as shown in Table 8.10 appears.

The critical t-value obtained in the printout is 0.002; i.e., the difference is significant on the 99.8% level. It is noted that the t-statistic (4.64) is different from the one calculated. This will be addressed below.

8.7 CHECKING THE MEANING OF PARAMETERS IN PROGRAMS: PROGRAM VALIDATION

Whenever a statistical (or other) program is being used, it is important (a) to validate it; i.e., does it give the "right" numbers with a variety of sets of data, where the numbers can be calculated by hand? (b) What, actually, do the various statements that are presented in the computer output mean?

8.7.1 EXAMPLE 8.3

Carry out an unpaired t-test for sets C and F.

TABLE 8.10. StatWorks™ Output.

Data File: Table 8.10

Independent Samples...

Variable:	Set B	Set E
Mean:	11.270000	10.262500
Std. Deviation:	0.370135	0.249583
Observations:	5	4

t-statistic:	4.635335	Hypothesis:
Degrees of Freedom:	7	Ho: $\mu1 = \mu2$
Significance:	0.002	Ha: $\mu1 \neq \mu2$

TABLE 8.11. Printout from StatWorks™.

Data File: Table 8.11
Independent Samples...

Variable:	Set C	Set F
Mean:	13.300000	12.460000
Std. Deviation:	0.595819	0.559464
Observations:	5	5

t-statistic:	2.298138	Hypothesis:
Degrees of Freedom:	8	Ho: $\mu 1 = \mu 2$
Significance:	0.051	Ha: $\mu 1 \neq \mu 2$

8.7.2 ANSWER 8.3

StatWorks™ gives the printout in Table 8.11. It is noted that

(1) The difference between the means is 0.84.

(2) The pooled variance is $(0.313 + 0.355)5/8 = 0.4175$ so that $s = 0.6461$.

(3) Hence, the t-value is $(0.84/0.6461)\sqrt{(25/10)} = 2.06$.

The reason that there is a slight difference between this number and the number obtained from the program is that the latter uses the following formula:

$$t = (X_1 - X_2)/[(s_1^2/n_1) + (s_2^2/n_2)]^{1/2} \qquad (8.15)$$

However, there is no way of knowing this other than by validation. The two formulae are identical if the two s-values are the same, but as they become more different, the more different are the s-values from the two sets. The Youden method [rather than the one in Equation (8.15)] is the preferred one, but the programmed method has the advantage of being easy to carry out.

It is noted from the output that the probability associated with the t-value of 2.298 is 5.1%. If a two-sided table is consulted, it is seen that 5% corresponds to a t of 2.306 (with 8 df), so that it is indeed a two-sided value that is used in the program as well.

8.8 UNEQUAL VARIANCES

If the variances are significantly different, then the sets do not come from the same population. One may still ask whether there is a significant difference between the means, and in this case Equation (8.12) is used, except the degrees of freedom are calculated by means of the formula:

$$\mathrm{df}' = [(s_1^2/n_1) + (s_2^2/n^2)]^2/[\{(s_1^2/n_1)^2/n_1\} + \{(s_2^2/n_2)^2/n_2\}] \qquad (8.16)$$

The use of this is rarer than in the cases cited above, where the variances did not differ significantly.

8.9 PAIRED *t*-TEST

As an example of a paired *t*-test, consider the data in Table 8.12. If the determinations are paired, e.g., if the values in sets A and B were comparable, i.e., the same assay but run one hour apart, so that 1 in sets A and B were the same sample, then a paired *t*-test can be carried out. This consists of taking the differences, *d,* of each determination (1–5), and stating that these differences are distributed like *t.* The standard deviation is simply the standard deviation of the values of *d.* The values of *d* have an average of 1.04 and an sem of 0.1623; hence, the true mean is in the interval:

$$d_{\mathrm{avg}} - \{(t_{1-\alpha,\nu})(\mathrm{sem})\} < \mu_d < d_{\mathrm{avg}} + \{(t_{1-\alpha,\nu})(\mathrm{sem})\} \qquad (8.17)$$

If $\mu = 0$ is included in this interval, then it may be concluded that the test fails to show a significant difference. In other words, if

$$t = d_{\mathrm{avg}} - 0/\mathrm{sem} > t_{1-\alpha,\nu} \qquad (8.18)$$

then there is a significant difference on the $100(1 - \alpha)\%$ level. The numbers in this case are such that

$$t = 1.04/0.1623 = 6.4 \qquad (8.19)$$

The table to be consulted is a one-sided test, since we are examining the probability of a difference being larger than something, rather than being

TABLE 8.12. Sets A and B from Table 8.1 Treated by Paired *t*-Testing.

Sample #	1	2	3	4	5
Assay A	10.50	10.45	10.10	10.00	10.10
Assay B	11.00	11.90	11.20	11.25	11.0
Difference	0.50	1.45	1.10	1.25	0.90

TABLE 8.13. Printout from StatWorks™.

Data File: Table 8.12
Paired Samples...

Variable:	Set A	Set B
Mean:	10.230000	11.270000
Std. Deviation:	0.228035	0.370135
Paired Observations: 5		

t-statistic:	-6.406827	Hypothesis:
Degrees of Freedom:	4	Ho: μ1 = μ2
Significance:	0.003	Ha: μ1 ≠ μ2

in an interval. Hence, the correct part (one-sided) of Appendix 3 must be consulted. In StatWorks™, the procedure is the same as above, except the circle indicating paired comparison is highlighted. The printout, in this case, is shown in Table 8.13. It is noted that the t-statistic is the same as calculated in Equation (8.19) ($t = 6.4$). The significance is 0.3%.

8.10 χ^2-TEST

The χ^2-test tests data for expected frequency or expected number of occurrences (E) against observed frequency or observed number of occurrences (O). The quantity

$$(O - E)^2/E \tag{8.20}$$

is distributed by χ^2. The number of degrees of freedom is a matter of the particular situation that is being considered.

8.10.1 CONTINGENCY TABLES

This approach was first used in the last century in evaluating treatment with vaccines, dividing populations into treated and nontreated groups, and observing, e.g., the incidences of infection and noninfection in treated groups and comparing these numbers with those in the untreated groups.

A pharmaceutical example would be the following: In a company, the tablet operation is a three-shift operation, and it is suspected that the operation differs by shift. To test this hypothesis, the hardnesses recorded on one product made on all the three shifts are monitored (from batch records of the past). The numbers are divided into three ranges: 4–6 kP (low or

TABLE 8.14. Example of Chi Square Test.

	Number of Batches.			
Hardness=	Low	Medium	High	Row Total
Night	34	20	20	74
Evening	30	50	40	120
Day	45	55	50	150
Column Totals	119	105	120	**344.**

"−"), 7–9 kP (medium or "o"), and 10–14 kP (high or "+"). Obviously, the number of batches may differ, and the results in Table 8.14 are recorded (the numbers indicating number of batches). The grand total then is 344.

The degree of freedom in a situation like this is (3 − 1) × (3 − 1). Table 8.15 is now constructed. If this is compared with χ^2 for 2 × 2 = 4 degrees of freedom, which is 9.5, it is seen that the value

$$(O - E)^2/E = 16.9 > 9.5 = \chi^2_{4.0.95} \tag{8.21}$$

is significant; i.e., there is a difference between the performance of the three shifts.

8.10.2 TEST FOR CURVATURE

Another example, pertinent to scientific studies, is the following. Suppose we are conducting scientific experiments, e.g., kinetic experiments,

TABLE 8.15. Data from Table 8.14 with Expected Values.

	O	E	$(O-E)^2/E$
N-	34	25.6	2.76
E-	30	41.5	3.19
D-	45	51.9	0.92
No	20	22.6	0.30
Eo	50	36.6	4.90
Do	55	45.8	1.85
N+	20	25.8	1.31
E+	40	41.9	0.86
D+	50	52.3	0.10
Total			16.9

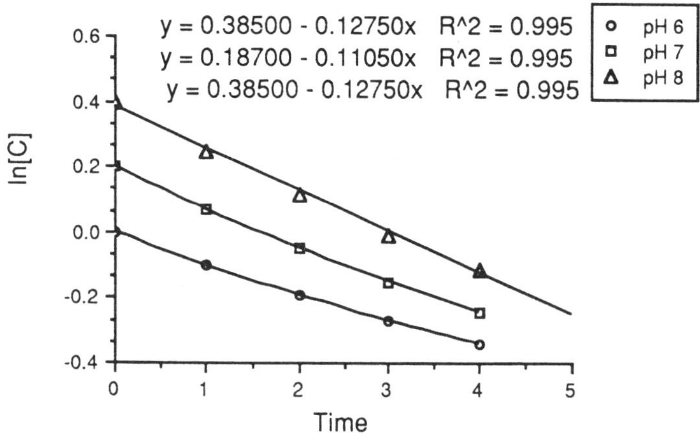

Figure 8.1 Example of kinetic data at three pH values. The two lower curves have been fit by interpolation, the upper curve by least squares fit.

where the values (e.g., concentrations), decrease in time, and assume that we plot the logarithm of the value (C) as a function of time. Suppose, also, that we always do at least four time points in each study. The curves for three experimental conditions, e.g., three pH values, could be as shown in Figure 8.1.

It is demonstrated in the upper curve of the graph that the first point is above the least squares fit line, the next three are below, and the last one is above. This is true for all the curves shown, and the two lower curves have been fit by interpolation and indicate that there is curvature. The question is whether this is really correct.

Suppose these data are part of a larger study (e.g., a pH profile) where fifty curves have been carried out (giving fifty rate constants). In this case, we may have drawn lines in all cases and wondered if the method is correct. We will assume that there are four, not five, points, and we can now divide the experimental space into four categories: initial (1) time, second time point (2), third (3), and last time points (4). We can then group the data by stating whether the experimental point was above (+) or below

TABLE 8.16. Contingency Table for Figure 8.1.

Totals	1	2	3	4	Row
High(+)	13	1	2	12	28
Low(-)	2	14	13	3	32
Column Totals	15	15	15	15	60

TABLE 8.17. Data from Table 8.16.

Condition	O	E	$(O-E)^2/E$
1+	13	7	5.14
1 -	2	8	4.50
2+	1	7	5.14
2 -	14	8	4.5
3+	2	7	3.57
3 -	13	8	3.13
4+	12	7	3.57
4 -	3	8	3.13
Total			32.58

(−) the line and obtain a contingency table (Table 8.16) where the bolded figure is the grand total.

The degrees of freedom are $(2 - 1) \times (4 - 1) = 3$. It is seen that the value

$$(O - E)^2/E = 32.58 > 12.84 = \chi^2_{3,0.995} \tag{8.22}$$

i.e., at a very high degree of significance. Hence, there is curvature in the data (Table 8.17), and another model would have to be sought. (This could be first-order kinetics with an equilibrium condition.)

8.11 THE WILCOXON/FRIEDMAN TEST

Sometimes, the fact that all the values in one set are lower than that in another or in other sets justifies the statement that the first set differs significantly from the remainder. If the data are (or can be) paired, then the Wilcoxon/Friedman (Wilcoxon, 1949) test is often appropriate.

The data are placed in tabular form in k columns (i.e., there are k sets) and ranked by assigning the number "1" to the smallest value and the number k to the largest value in each line (comparative determination). The sums of the ranks, T, may be transformed in a fashion so as to make them distributed by χ^2:

$$\chi^2 = [\{12/nk(k + 1)\} \times \Sigma T^2] - 3n(k + 1) \tag{8.23}$$

with $k - 1$ degrees of freedom. This is best illustrated by example.

8.11.1 EXAMPLE 8.4

The assays in Table 8.12 were obtained by assaying a solution of a drug substance by five different assay procedures. Use Equation (8.23) to establish significance.

8.11.2 ANSWER 8.4

The data are shown with ranking in Table 8.18. It is seen that, if two sets have the same number, then the rank is "split" (sample 2, C and D). The parameter in Equation (7.10) is calculated:

$$\chi^2 = [\{12/nk(k + 1)\} \times \Sigma T^2] - 3n(p + 1)$$

$$= \{12/(6 \times 5 \times 6)\} \times (21^2 + 12^2 + 23.5^2$$

$$+ 27.5^2 + 6^2) - (18 \times 6) = 128.6 - 108 = 20.6$$

The df is equal to the number of columns (items being compared) minus one. Since

$$\chi^2_{0.995} = 20.6 > \chi^2_{0.995} = 14.86$$

it follows that there is a significant difference in the set. Visual inspection would suggest that assay method E gives significantly smaller numbers than the other methods. (One should, however, not "discard" *E* as being "invalid." It *could* be the only one that gives an accurate number.)

8.12 EQUIVALENCE TESTING

The GMP guidelines caused the FDA, in 1972, to issue biopharmaceutics guidelines. If a formula of a product is changed substantially or if a company conducts clinical studies on a product and compares the blood

TABLE 8.18. Assays of Several Samples by Different Procedures A–E.

Sample	A	Rank	B	Rank	C	Rank	D	Rank	E	Rank
1	1.38	5	1.30	2	1.31	3	1.36	4	1.11	1
2	1.33	3	1.29	2	1.34	4.5	1.34	4.5	1.22	1
3	1.33	3	1.30	2	1.36	4	1.40	5	1.16	1
4	1.36	3	1.25	2	1.40	5	1.38	4	1.24	1
5	1.35	4	1.24	2	1.34	3	1.39	5	1.19	1
6	1.29	3	1.28	2	1.35	4	1.38	5	1.14	1
Rank Totals:		21		12		23.5		27.5		6

TABLE 8.19. Blood Levels (mg/ml) after Oral Administration of Two Products.

Time(hours)	1	2	4	8	12
Set A (mg/L)	15	20	12	5	3
Set B (mg/L)	25	21	18	5.5	3.5

level data of theirs to that of a competitor, then there must, by necessity, be a comparison between a set A and a set B.

It would be convenient if such a test would result in A = B, but as we have seen, it is not possible to achieve that. Instead, it is only possible to achieve the statement that the testing performed failed to show a difference between A and B.

If a test was conducted where each patient was his own control, i.e., he was given first A, then a placebo, then B, and blood levels tested, then, in a small trial, the results in Table 8.19 might result.

If a paired *t*-test is carried out, then the significance (StatWorks™, descriptive, *t*-test, paired) is 0.132; i.e., one may only state with 86.8% confidence that the data are different. A Wilcoxon-Friedman test would give a better percentage.

The original official requirement for two products to be equivalent was that they not be significantly different on the 95% confidence level and that the test is set up so that a true difference of 5% is detectable. This requirement was later changed.

8.13 THE POWER OF A TEST

In a *t*-test, we have seen that one calculates a difference between means (dif) and a 95% (or other confidence limit), q, about the difference; i.e., one concludes that if

$$\text{dif} - q_{\alpha=0.05} > 0$$

then one may say with better than 95% confidence that zero is not in the interval and that, hence, there is a significant difference. At a higher level of confidence (e.g., 97.5%), this may also be true, but at an even higher level of confidence (e.g., 99%), it may not be true, i.e.,

$$\text{dif} > q_{\alpha=0.05} > 0$$

$$\text{dif} > q_{\alpha=0.025} > 0$$

$$\text{dif} < q_{\alpha=0.01} > 0$$

The point where the dif and q-values are equal is the number printed out in the program runs shown above.

8.14 TEST FOR NORMALITY

It is often of importance to know whether sets of data are distributed normally, given, for instance, the following situation: samples of a new product have been tested for dissolution and the Q_{45} figures obtained. (These are the percent of label claim released after 45 minutes in the dissolution test.) It would be desirable to know whether variations in these figures are due to content uniformity. The results for a given product, expressed as %LC, were obtained and are shown in Table 8.20. When the last three columns are pooled, the figures in the bottom cell result.

If the data are placed in StatWorks™, then one may conduct t-tests, for instance, to see if all had dissolved. In essence, if the average is taken of the last three columns, then if a t-test fails to show a significant difference between the Q_{45}-value and the uniformity value, it may be concluded that "all the drug in the dosage form has dissolved at 45 minutes."

The question might be raised whether the data are normally distributed. Here we shall lump all the "uniformity of dosage form" data, i.e., obtain

TABLE 8.20. Q_{45}-Values and Content Uniformity Values (%LC).

Unit #	Q_{45}-Value	Content Uniformity Results		
1	97.7	99.6	95.4	97.0
2	105.2	110.2	105.0	94.7
3	105	96.1	95.8	103.5
4	107.8	92.1	96.4	95.4
5	99.8	95.7	92.4	95.1
6	94.0	95.4	96.7	94.8
7	94.7	106.9	94.8	94.7
8	95.2	96.0	96.7	94.6
9	98.3	96.8	93.2	95.2
10	104.2	115.7	96.2	94.9
11	94.3			
12	95.5			
Content Uniformity:				
N:			30	
Mean:			97.6	
Standard Deviation:			5.37	
SEM:			0.98	

a total of thirty numbers. StatWorks™ can test this for normality, and if this is done, the result will show:

- statistic: 0.342026
- significance: 0.031

The question is: What do these numbers signify? StatWorks™, under DATA, has an address stating SORT, and it is possible to pool all the data in the last three columns and then sort this column.

Sturges's rule states that, for normality, one should use n intervals, given by

$$n = 1 + 3.322 \log_{10} [n] = 1 + 3.322 \cdot 1.48 = 5.9 = 6$$

It is noted that the range is 92 to 116, so that the interval length should be $(116 - 92)/6 = 4$. If this is done, then the intervals and the number of occurrences will be as shown in Table 8.21.

It is obvious, from simply looking at the figures, that they are not normally distributed. But for the sake of exercise, the execution of the normality test, as it is normally carried out, is shown below.

The standard deviation is 5.34 and the mean is 97.6, so the intervals in Table 8.21 may be shown as a deviation from the mean in terms of standard deviations, and this is given in Table 8.22. Table 8.23 is then constructed from Table 8.21.

There are eight intervals, so the degrees of freedom (Daniels, 1978) are $8 - 2 = 6$. For six degrees of freedom, and the χ^2-table in Appendix 8 will simply show that the probability for a value of 20.1 is less than 0.5%.

The statistics used in the StatWorks™ program are, therefore, different from that used above. The fact is clear that the "significance" implied is the probability of the data actually being normal; i.e., the probability is fairly low (3%).

TABLE 8.21. Data from Table 8.20.

Interval	No of Occurrences
92-95.99	16
96 - 99.99	9
100 -103.99	1
104 - 107.99	2
108 - 111.99	1
112 - 116	1

TABLE 8.22. Data from Table 8.21.

Number	Deviation from Mean	Expressed in Terms of SD's	Area Under Normal Curve	Expected Fraction in Interval
<92				
				0.147
92	-5.6	-1.05	0.147	
				0.235
96	-1.6	-0.30	0.382	
				0.310
100	2.4	0.50	0.692	
				0.193
104	6.4	1.20	0.885	
				0.089
108	10.4	1.95	0.974	
				0.023
112	14.4	2.70	0.997	
				0.003
116	18.4	3.45	1.000	
				0.000
>116				
Total				1.000

TABLE 8.23. Data from Table 8.19.

Interval	No of Occurrences N	Fraction Expected	No of Occurrences Expected F	$\frac{(N-F)^2}{F}$
<92	0	0.147	4.41	4.41
92-95.99	16	0.235	7.05	11.36
96 - 99.99	9	0.310	9.30	0.01
100 -103.99	1	0.193	5.79	3.96
104 - 107.99	2	0.089	2.67	0.17
108 - 111.99	1	0.023	0.69	0.14
112 - 116	1	0.003	0.09	0
>116	0	0	0	
Total				20.05

8.15 PROBLEMS

(1) A company decides to submit a drug product to the FDA. They perform a biobatch clinical trial to show equivalence. The drug is administered orally, blood levels are determined at different times after administration, and the data are as follows:

		Blood Levels, mg/L		
Time hrs.	Patient No.	Original Trial Batch	Patient No.	Large Biobatch
1	A	15.2	G	10.5
1	B	20.0	H	19.9
1	C	13.1	J	12.5
1	D	12.2	K	12.1
1	E	19.2	L	9.1
1	F	17.7	M	17.2
2	A	35.2	G	35.0
2	B	40.5	H	40.0
2	C	36.1	J	35.2
2	D	35.2	K	36.9
2	E	37.2	L	30.0
2	F	31.7	M	37.2

(For simplicity, only two time points are considered. In real situations, more likely, eight time points of the blood level curve would be taken into account.) What is the best manner of deciding whether there is a significant difference between the original batch and the biobatch?

If, instead of this being a biobatch compared with an old batch, it were a small batch made like the old batch, being compared at the same time with a large-scale biobatch, and if patients G–M were equal to patients A–F (i.e., each patient first got the small batch, then later the large batch), what test should be applied?

(2) Four different assay methods are used on four preparations of the same product; i.e., four aliquots are drawn from a stock solution and assayed by the four methods and likewise with three other stock solutions.

Perform an *F*-test. Are there other tests that could be employed?

No.	Assay Method 1	Assay Method 2	Assay Method 3	Assay Method 4
1	15.8	15.7	15.5	15.5
2	15.5	15.7	15.2	15.5
3	15.9	15.3	15.1	15.5
4	15.6	15.1	15.4	15.8

(3) A graduate scientist has performed assays of furoic acid in solid samples of various degrees of decomposition. The method is spectrophotometric. The decomposition product is measured at another wavelength. The following assays are obtained, where the sets of three are independent and where the decomposition assay corresponds to the parent compound assay (e.g., 15 and 0.1 were obtained from the same aliquot):

Storage Time (months)	0	1	2
Furoic Acid (mmoles)/ml	15,14.9,15.1	12.1,12.0,12.5	10,9.9,10.2
Decomposition (mmoles)/ml	0.1,0.1,0.0	3.0,2.5,2.8	4.0,3.9,4.1

What conclusion can be drawn?

(4) An assay is tested in the presence and in the absence of potassium chloride. Following are results of quadruplicate assays of a given sample:

With KCl	75.5	75.9	76.2	75.1
Without KCl	80.2	82	78	85

Devise a significance test and calculate whether there is a significant difference between the numbers. Can a paired t-test be used?

8.16 ANSWERS

(1) The data are entered into a StatWorks™ program and an unpaired t-test is carried out for original versus 1 hour, with the α-fractional probabilities shown below. A Wilcoxon signed rank test is also carried out with the program and gives the following percentages:

Test	Original/Bio 1 hour	Original/Bio 2 hour
Unpaired t-test	0.24	0.553
Wilcoxon Rank	0.014	0.173

The rank test is much more meaningful in this case and shows a significant difference (on the 98.6% confidence level) for the one-hour point between the original batch and the biobatch.

(2) The totals and the variances are listed on the following page.

Sample #	Assay Method 1	Assay Method 2	Assay Method 3	Assay Method 4	Sums
Totals, T	62.8	61.8	61.2	62.3	GT=248.1
Variance	0.0333	0.0900	0.0333	0.0225	0.1791
$T^2/4$	985.96	954.81	936.36	970.3225	3847.4525

$$s_b^2 = (1/3)(3847.4525 - [248.1^2/16]) = 0.351875/\underline{3} = 0.1173$$

$$s_w^2 = 3(0.1791)/\underline{12} = 0.044775$$

$$\text{Variance ratio} = 0.1173/0.044775 = 2.62 < 3.49 = F_{crit}(3,12)$$

Hence, the F-test fails to show a significant difference between the sets. If, however, an unpaired t-test is performed between assay 1 and 3, the difference is significant on the 98% level. It is concluded that assay 3 gives a lower assay than method 1. One could then run t-tests to show that they fail to show differences between the other assay methods. Note that if one test fails and another is significant, then it is the latter that counts.

(3) If it is only furoic acid decomposing to one decomposition product, then the total number of moles of the two should be unaltered as a function of time (mass balance). The totals are shown below:

Sum of Furoic Acid and Decomposition Product

Sample #	Time 0	Time 1	Time 2
1	15.1	15.1	14.0
2	15.0	14.5	12.9
3	15.1	15.3	14.3

These have been subjected to unpaired and paired t-tests below, and it is seen that there is a significant difference between the two-month sample and both the initial (unpaired) and the one-month (paired).

Test	Comparison	α-Value
Unpaired t-test	0/2	0.035
Unpaired t-test	1/2	0.065
Paired t-test	1/2	0.022

Hence, it may be concluded (on at least the 96.5% confidence level) that there is not mass balance at the two-month point. The reason for this may be manyfold (evaporation or further decomposition of the decomposition product).

(4) A paired t-test cannot be used, since the solutions assayed are not the same in the two groups.

StatWorks™ unpaired t-test gives the following results:

Descriptive:

$$x_{1,\mathrm{avg}} = 75.675 \qquad x_{2,\mathrm{avg}} = 82.3$$

i.e.,

$$\text{difference} = d = 5.625$$

$$s_1^2 = 0.229 \qquad s_1^2 = 8.75$$

t-test (StatWorks™):

$$\alpha = 0.009$$

That is, there is a significant difference on the 99% level.

It was shown earlier that StatWorks™ uses the formula

$$t_{\nu,1-\alpha}[(s_1^2/n_1) + (s_2^2/n^2)]^{1/2}$$

In this example, this would be 3.707 × 1.50 = 5.57; i.e., the mean would be in the interval

$$5.625 \pm 5.57 \text{ just barely} > \text{zero on the 99\% level } (\alpha = 0.01)$$

This is in accordance with the program that gave $\alpha = 0.009$. However, the variance ratio is $8.75/0.229 = 38.2 \gg 28.24$, which is the critical F-value on the 99% level. Hence, the degrees of freedom should be calculated according to Equation (8.16).

The fact that the variances differ shows that there is a significant difference between the two methods. But are the actual assay numbers "different"?

The easiest manner to approach this formula is to calculate the s/n terms:

$$s_1^2/n_1 = 0.229/4 = 0.05725; \qquad s_2^2/n_2 = 8.764 = 2.19$$

$$(s_1^2/n_1)^2/n_1 = 0.05725^2/4 = 0.00083$$

$$(s_2^2/n_2)^2/n_2 = 2.19^2/4 = 1.199$$

TABLE 9.1. Assays of "Previous" Batches of a Product for Which a Sampling Scheme Is Sought.

Batch—>	1	2	3	Totals
	100	101	101.5	
	98	98.5	100	
	99.3	100	99.5	
s^2	1.03	1.583	1.083	
SS	2.06	3.17	2.17	7.4
df	2	2	2	6

TABLE 9.2. Program for Calculation of Upper and Lower Limit.

```
100  INPUT "Standard Deviation="; S
110  INPUT "Degrees of Freedom="; D
120  INPUT "Lower Specification Limit="; L
130  INPUT "Highest N=";M
140  PRINT "N", "Delta", "Lower Limit"
130  PRINT "__________________"
210  IF N = 3 GOTO 215
215  T = 2.92
220  GOTO 225
225  IF N = 4 GOTO 230
230  T = 2.35
235  GOTO 240
240  IF N = 5 GOTO 245
245  T = 2.13
250  GOTO 255
255  IF N = 6 GOTO 260
260  T = 2.02
265  IF N = 7 GOTO 270
270  T = 1.94
275  IF N = 8 GOTO 280
280  T = 1.89
290  GOTO 300
300  FOR N = 2 TO M STEP 1
400  y1 = S/D
410  y2 = y1^(.5)
430  y3 = y2*2.2
440  y4 = N^(.5)
450  y5 = (y3/y4)
460  y6 = T*y5
PRINT N,y6, L+y6
NEXT N
```

It is noted that LPRINT may have to be substituted for PRINT with some printers.

TABLE 9.3. Calculation of Number of Samples to Assay.

N	$t_{N-1,0.9}$(1)	∂ SD=1.111	Lowest Spec.
2	1.73	3.27	98.3
2	1.41	1.67	97.7
4	1.22	2.31	97.3
5	1.09	2.06	97.1
6	1.00	1.89	96.9

for $N = 6$ and a lower limit of 95%, with the standard deviation of 1.111 then the printout is shown in Table 9.3.

A comment on the last column: If it is desired to state, with 95% confidence, that the assay number is (truly) above 95% label claim, then the lowest "in-house" specification limit would have to be $95 + 1.50 = 96.5$% label claim, if, for instance, the sample size were $N = 3$. If the sample size were six, then the lowest in-house specification limit would be $95 + 0.9 = 95.9$ and so on.

9.2 SAMPLING BY ATTRIBUTES

The most important examples of sampling by attributes in pharmaceutics are (a) blending validation and (b) the USP content uniformity test. The aspect of blending was covered in Section 7.7 and is associated with the binomial distribution. Some of the pertinent properties are repeated here for convenience.

Given a population with a fraction, p, of drug (probability of success), if a sample of size N (N particles, N tries) is taken, then the probability of picking a sample with x drug particles (successes) is

$$\Pr(x) = \begin{bmatrix} N \\ x \end{bmatrix} p^x(1 - p)^{N-x} \tag{9.2}$$

where $\begin{bmatrix} N \\ x \end{bmatrix}$ is the number of ways in which x articles can be removed from N articles. It is given by the binomial formula:

$$\begin{bmatrix} N \\ x \end{bmatrix} = N!/((N - x)!x!) \tag{9.3}$$

The average number is

$$\text{avg}\,(x) = Np \tag{9.4}$$

and the standard deviation is

$$\text{var}(x) = p(1 - p)/N \tag{9.5}$$

In the sampling progams, if one samples by attributes, i.e., if there are two possible events—a reject or a good sample—so-called operational characteristics curves will result.

One talks about consumer's risk and manufacturer's cost. The former is the probability of a defective batch being accepted, and the latter is the probability of a satisfactory batch being rejected. The level of defects is a matter of the particular situation. A manufacturer may state that 5% defects is the acceptable quality control level (AQL), and that he wants only a 10% probability of rejecting (90% of passing) a batch with less defects; on the other hand, 10% is the largest number of defects he really wants to see on the market (AOQL = acceptable outgoing quality level), and he then wants only a 10% probability of passing such a batch.

There are many curves that will pass through each of these points on an AQL curve, and a couple of such curves are shown in Figure 9.1, where the acceptable level is zero or one defect in samples of N.

9.3 A PHARMACEUTICAL EXAMPLE

The USP applies a content uniformity test in which thirty (solid dosage form) units (i.e., capsules or tablets) are taken at random from a batch and ten are assayed. The USP defines a unit containing 85–115% of label claim as a "good" unit, units between 75 and 85% and between 115 and 125% of label claim are minor defects, and units below 75% and above 125% of label claim are major defects. The ruling is that, if any of the samples

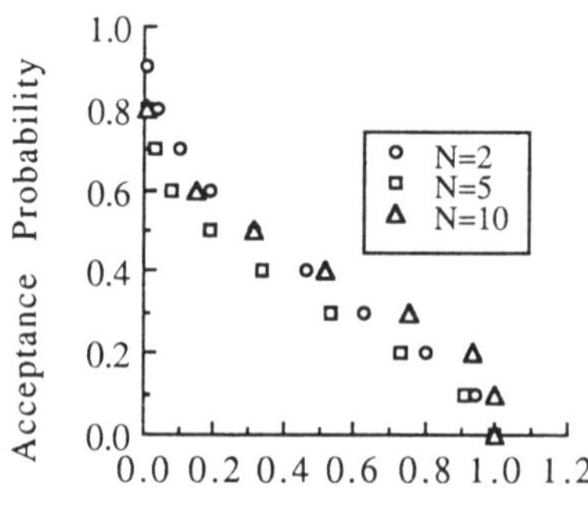

Figure 9.1 Operational characteristics chart for various sampling schemes.

tested are major defects, then the batch is ruled unacceptable (rejectable). If, in the first sampling of ten, there is more than one minor defect, then the batch is also rejected. If there is one minor defect, then the remaining twenty units are assayed, and of the thirty units, only one may be a minor defect (and none may be major). In the 1985 issue of the USP, a further restriction was imposed; viz., the relative standard deviation could be no more than 6% at the first sampling of ten units. The USP content uniformity test essentially considers units below 85% and above 115% as defects.[13] In a sample of thirty, only one defect may be present, so that only a fraction of 0.033 may lie outside these limits, 0.016 below 85% and 0.016 above 115%. If one considers the contents as being normally distributed, then an area of 0.016 corresponds to 2.1 standard deviations. Hence, 15% corresponds to 2.1 standard deviations, so that one may consider the USP content uniformity criterion to be associated with a standard deviation of 15/2.1 = 7.1 RSD.[14] If one now considers the principles of sampling by variance, then the average assay has a 95% confidence limit ($1 - \alpha = 0.95$) of

$$\pm t_{N-1,(1-\alpha)} s/\sqrt{N} \qquad (9.6)$$

One might now ask: what does the test consider a practical limit for the average assay? Considering that $t_{0.05,9} = 2.2622$, one may calculate that

$$2.2622 \times 7.1/\sqrt{10} = 4.8\% = 5\% \qquad (9.7)$$

so that the USP considers an interval for an average to be 95–105%.

9.4 BLENDING VALIDATION

In a recent decision by the courts (the Bahr decision), it was ruled that, to assure that a product is sufficiently well blended (blending validation), the sample size must equal, at most, three times the dose size; i.e., if a batch of powder is made for 1,000,000 capsules, each of a fill weight of 300 mg, then the largest sample can be no more than 900 mg. As in the "content uniformity" for the final product, ten samples are taken, and aside from the actual assays having to be within limits, the allowed standard deviation on the sample is 5% (as judged by statements in the Pink Sheet). The problem lies in the problem of obtaining a representative sample.

[13]The distinction between major and minor defect has no bearing on the considerations here.
[14]This is slightly different from the population standard deviation of 10% alleged to be the basis for the USP content uniformity test.

Samples are taken by a "thief" (a long hollow rod of two concentric cylinders, one inside the other). In the act of taking the sample, the powder blend is disturbed and there have been numerous examples where a powder "failed" validation, but the tablets or capsules produced were satisfactory.

The restriction of the sample size is a product of the lack of scientific understanding on the part of the court. It is obvious that, if one desired to know the standard deviation of a sample of m grams, one could take M grams and simply multiply the standard deviation from the M grams with $(M/m)^{1/2}$. This is only strictly true for "completely" blended powder samples, i.e., samples that have reached their final, random standard deviation [given by Equation (9.5)]. Monte Carlo methods (Carstensen, 1993), however, demonstrate that, for nearly completely blended samples, this is also true.

9.5 CONTROL CHARTS

The Good Manufacturing Practices require that sampling be random, but many (in fact, most) pharmaceutical sampling plans are not random, but rather stratified. This comes from the fact that much in-processing work is done by control charts. Samples of tablets may, for instance, be collected every 30 minutes and checked for weight and hardness and the data entered in a control chart. Collected samples may then be pooled and sampled randomly from the pool, or the entire pool may be the sample. This, however, is *not* random sampling. In a way, it is more meaningful sampling, but it is reemphasized that it is not random.

The workings of a control chart are best illustrated by example. Table 9.4 shows the tablet weights of a product as it is made on the tablet machine. Samples of four are taken every hour and recorded.

Each sample is associated with (a) a range, R, and (b) a mean, x_{avg}. These must lie between certain limits given by the sought average ($x_{grand\text{-}avg}$) and a theoretical range, which is the expected standard deviation, s, times a factor. In reality, when a first batch is run, the grand average, X_{avg}, of the process is determined, and the average of the observed ranges, R_{avg}, is determined and the upper and lower control limits for the process determined by the following formula:

$$\text{UCL} = X_{avg} \pm A_1 R$$

where the values of A are given in Table 9.5. The ranges must lie in the following interval:

TABLE 9.4. In-Process Control Tablet Weights as a Function of Sampling Time.

Time (hours)	Average Weight (N=4) (mg)	Standard Deviation of Subsample (mg)	Range of Subsample (mg)
1	270.800	1.131	3.8
2	271.000	1.292	4.7
3	270.600	1.393	3.2
4	272.200	1.192	3.9
5	270.800	1.342	4.7
6	271.200	1.063	3.0
7	270.500	1.371	5.4
8	270.000	1.449	6.4
9	272.000	0.906	2.2
10	271.900	0.837	1.7
11	271.100	1.072	3.0
12	270.400	1.304	4.8
Averages	271.04		3.90

TABLE 9.5. Factors for Control Chart.

Size of Subgroup	Factors for Average	Factors for Range	
	A_1	A_2	A_3
2	1.880	0	3.267
3	1.023	9	4.358
4	0.729	0	4.698
5	0.577	0	4.918
6	0.483	0	5.078
7	0.419	0.076	5.203
8	0.373	0.136	5.307
9	0.297	0.184	5.397
10	0.308	0.223	5.469

$$\mathrm{LCL}_{\mathrm{range}} = A_2 R_{\mathrm{avg}} \tag{9.8}$$

$$\mathrm{UCL}_{\mathrm{range}} = A_3 R_{\mathrm{avg}} \tag{9.9}$$

where the values of A_2 and A_3 are shown in Table 9.5.

The control limits for the averages are therefore

$$\mathrm{UCL}_{\mathrm{avg}} = 271 + (0.729 \times 3.9) = 273.84 \tag{9.10}$$

and

$$\mathrm{LCL}_{\mathrm{avg}} = 271 - (0.729 \times 3.9) = 268.16 \tag{9.11}$$

These limits and the data from Table 9.4 are shown in Figure 9.2.

It can be seen that the control chart for the range should be

$$\mathrm{LCL} = 0 \tag{9.12}$$

$$\mathrm{UCL}_{\mathrm{range}} = 2.282 \times 3.9 = 8.9 \tag{9.13}$$

These data are shown in Figure 9.3.

It might, on the surface, seem that the use of the range as a measure of "limits" (rather than, for instance, using a standard deviation) is fallacious. However, even in a limited set of data as the one presented here, there is a correlation, as shown in Figure 9.4.

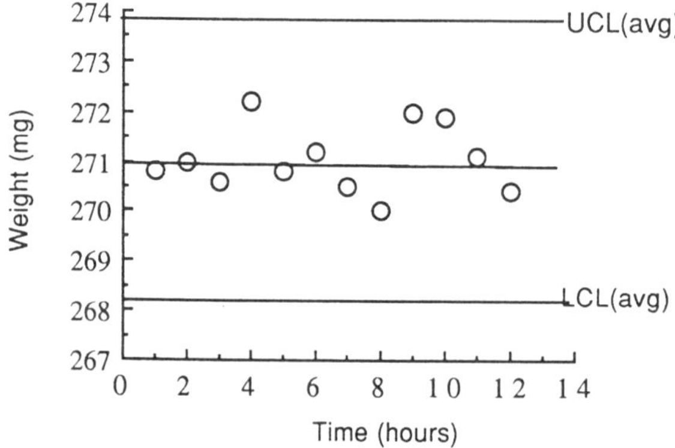

Figure 9.2 Data from Table 9.4 treated by Equations (9.8) to (9.11).

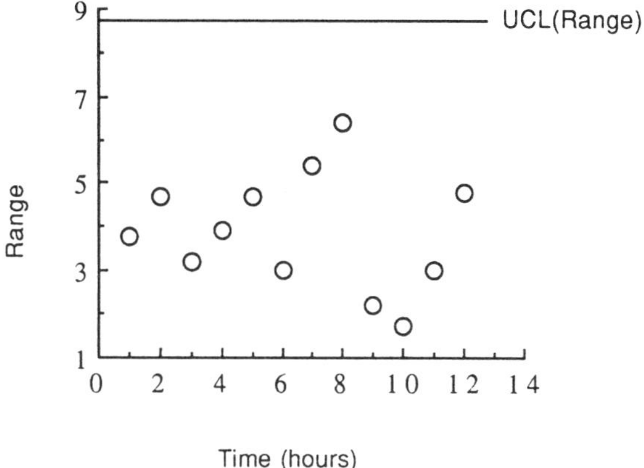

Figure 9.3 Data from Table 9.4 treated by Equation (9.13).

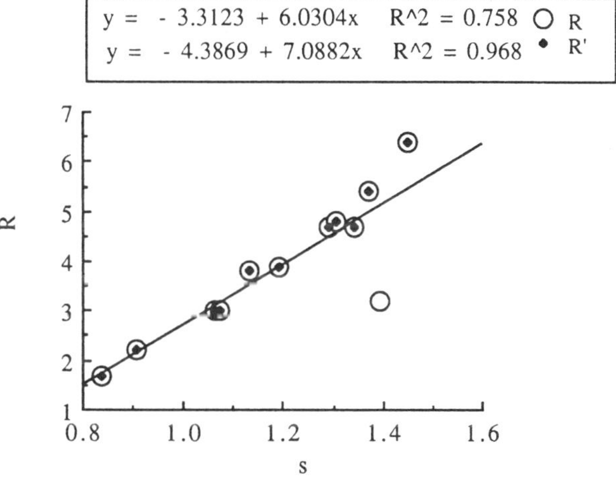

Figure 9.4 Graph of data from Table 9.4 showing correlation between range and standard deviation.

9.6 ARBITRARY AND TABULATED SAMPLE SIZES

Aside from the sampling schemes listed in the USP for dissolution testing (a sequential attribute scheme) and content uniformity, there are other, general rules for given circumstances.

When raw material is received by a pharmaceutical company, it is conventional to *square root sample.* This means that, if a shipment consists of ten drums, then three drums ($\sqrt{10}$) will be sampled.

The other preset type of sampling is that of the *military standards.* These are usually applied to government contracts and apply the principle that there are three levels of sampling: *reduced, normal,* and *tightened.* The level of sampling is decided contractually and would presumably depend on (a) the product, (b) the rating of the company, and/or (c) the critical nature of the quality of the product when used. Tables are available and are, for pharmaceutical batch sizes, of the order shown in Table 9.6.

Special considerations also apply in pre-DNA situations where GMP requirements (e.g., regarding retention samples) dictate numbers of samples differing from those in Table 9.6.

9.7 PROBLEMS

(1) Express Table 9.6 in equation form.

TABLE 9.6. Sample Size as a Function of Batch Size.

Batch Size	Average (B) Batch Size	Sample Size, S: Normal or Tightened (A)	Reduced (A)
91-150	120	20	8
151-280	215	32	13
2181-500	390	50	20
501-1200	850	80	32
1200-3200	2,200	125	80
3201-10,000	6,600	200	80
10,00-35,000	22,000	315	125
35,001-100,000	92,500	500	200
100,000-500,000	325,000	800	315

(2) If a dosage form contains 1000 particles and the drug content is 30%, give an expression for the probability of having a tablet with thirty-one drug particles.

(3) If Sterling's approximation formula is used, will the result be reasonable? Sterling's approximation formula is

$$\ln [N!] = N \ln [N] - N$$

If need be, write a program for the evaluation of the expression in Problem 9.2.

9.8 ANSWERS

(1) The data from the last two columns, when plotted versus the data in the second column give the following relationship:

Reduced: $\log s = 0.43 + 0.38 \log B$

Normal and tightened: $\log s = 0.83 + 0.38 \log B$

(2) $P(31) = [1000_{31}]0.3^{31}0.7^{969}$

(3) $= 1000!/(31! \times 935!)$ so

$$\ln [1000_{31}] = 1000 \ln [1000] - 1000 - 31 \ln [31] + 31$$
$$- 935 \ln [935] + 935 = 1000 \ln [1000] - 31 \ln [31]$$
$$935 \ln [935]$$

hence $\ln [P(31)]$ = this number $- 31 \ln [0.3] - 969 \ln [0.7]$

A simple calculation program in BASIC would be as follows:

```
100 Y1 = 1000*LOG(1000)
110 Y2 = 31*LOG(31)
120 Y3 = 969*LOG(969)
130 Y4 = Y1 - Y2 - Y3
150 X1 = 31*LOG(.3)
160 X2 = 969*LOG(.7)
170 Z = X1 + X2 + Y4
180 PRINT Z
```

which, when run, gives ln $[P] = -245$; i.e., $P(30)$ is a miniscule number. It should be pointed out that Sterling's formula is not necessarily a very good approximation formula. The point is that *individual* probabilities are very small.

9.9 REFERENCES

Bennett, C. A., and Franklin, N. L., (1954), *Statistical Analysis in Chemistry and the Chemical Industry.* John Wiley and Sons, Inc., New York.

Carstensen, J. T., (1993), *Drug Development and Industrial Pharmacy,* 19(20).

CHAPTER 10

Least Squares Fitting

A large number of data situations result in a linear presentation, and this chapter deals with the statistical methods for approaching this.

10.1 EQUATION FOR A STRAIGHT LINE

The usual nomenclature for the equation for a straight line is

$$y = a + bx \tag{10.1}$$

It is trivial, but needs to be stated in any event, that it takes at least two points (Figure 10.1) to define a straight line and that from two points $[(x_1, y_1)$ and $(x_2, y_2)]$, one may calculate the slope as

$$b = (y_1 - y_2)/(x_1 - x_2) \tag{10.2}$$

and the intercept may then be calculated from

$$(y - y_2) = b(x - x_2) \tag{10.3}$$

or the same expression using subscripts 1, rather than 2.

It stands to reason that, if one has only two points, then one really does not know if one is, indeed, dealing with a straight line.

With more than two points, one has some "feeling" for whether the points lie on a line, and from an intuitive point of view, the degree of freedom is therefore the number of points, n, minus two.

TABLE 10.1. Experimental versus Theoretical Stability Data.

Time	Theory	Experimental
0	1	1
3	0.99	0.989
6	0.98	0.975
9	0.97	0.969

10.2 CONCEPT OF LEAST SQUARES FITTING

The data in Table 10.1 will be used as an example in the following. They are data of a straight theoretical line (column 2). The last column consists of the same data set, but with an error imposed on each point.

The theoretical line is shown graphically in Figure 10.1, and the equation for the line is obtained and it is seen that the intercept is 100 and the slope = −0.33, i.e.,

$$y = 100 - 0.33x \tag{10.4}$$

As mentioned, the scatter is unknown.

Suppose we had a larger set of data, where the results were obtained with absolute precision; then the curve might look as shown in Figure 10.2. It is noted that the equation is the same as in Equation (10.4).

It is virtually impossible to obtain data this precise, and more

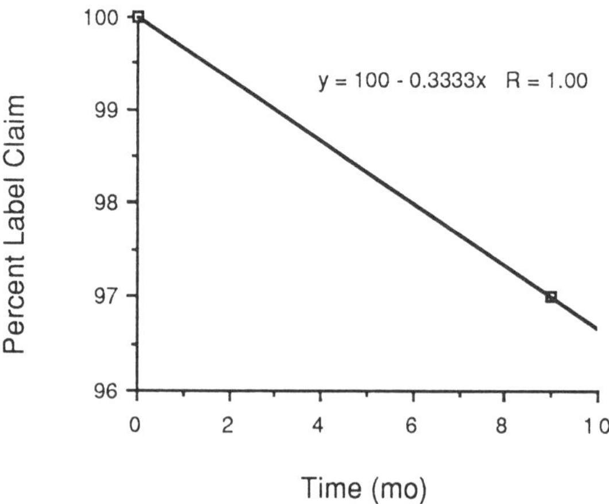

Figure 10.1 Example line through two points. Only one line can be drawn through two points. There is no sense of scatter (and order of reaction in case the data, as indicated, refer to a stability problem).

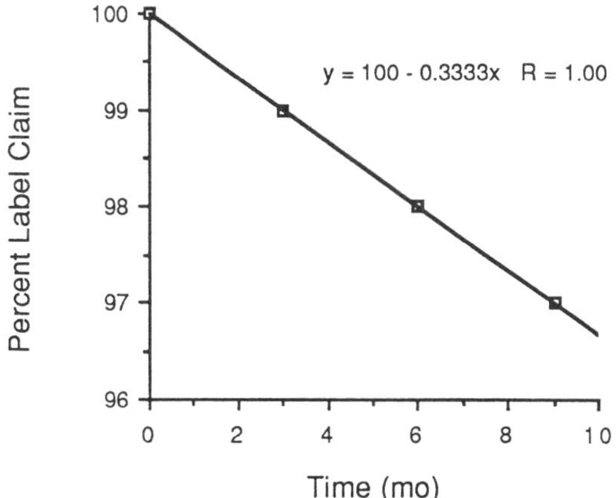

Figure 10.2 More points than in Figure 10.1 and exceedingly precise data.

realistically, let us assume that the data obtained were as shown in column 3 of Table 10.1 and Figure 10.3. These are, in essence, data obtained from Equation (10.4) but placing a random error on each point.

The (more realistic) data from the third column are shown in Figure 10.3 as simple points. In graphing, one does not, or course, simply connect the points (Figure 10.4). Such treatment is only applicable to cases like clinical temperature charts. This may seem self-evident, but such practices are still to be found in the pharmaceutical scientific literature. The treatment is not even realistic with a temperature chart because the temperature does not change abruptly at each point the temperature is recorded.

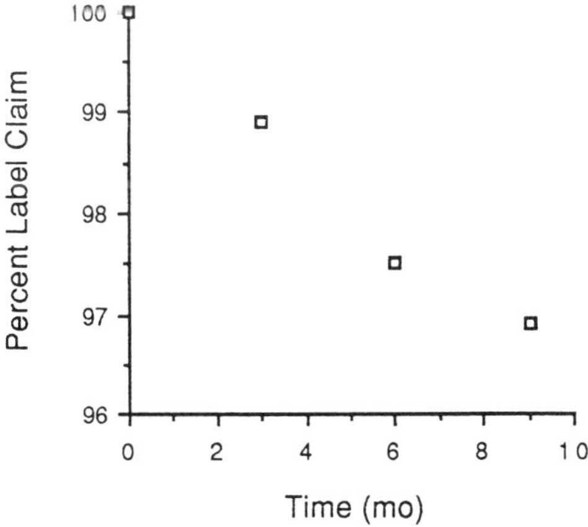

Figure 10.3 This figure shows the situation with more realistic data. The points scatter.

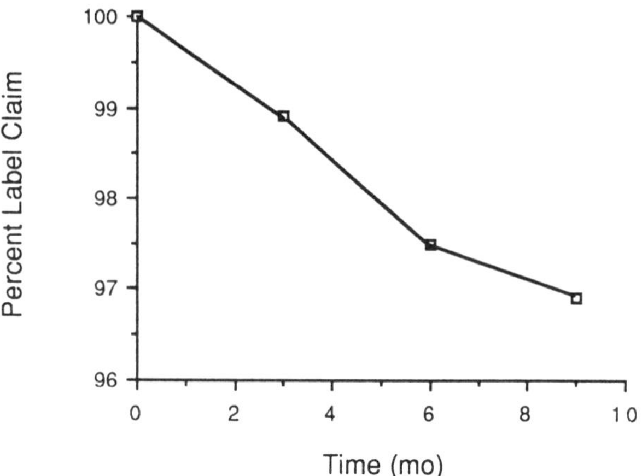

Figure 10.4 Improper treatment of the data in Figure 10.3.

One might then ask: How should one draw a *curve* through such points? First of all, it has to be decided from knowledge of the physical situation, whether the curve, indeed, could have nondifferential points (nicks) in it, but usually, this is not the case.

What type of differentiable curve would then be best fit to describe the data? In most circumstances of the above nature, the first attempt would be a straight line.

The question, then, is: What line should be drawn? One might pick a line one thought "reasonable," but two persons could draw two different lines, as shown in Figure 10.5.

From a colloquial point of view one might then ask which line is "better." For such decisions (as for all decisions in life), there must be a rule, and in this case the rule is that there exists a line (and we shall see later that it is one and only one line, i.e., *the* line) that possesses the quality that, when one calculates the distances from the experimental points to the line (Δ) and squares each of these (Δ^2) and sums these ($\Sigma\Delta^2$), then the line that has the least sum of squares, i.e., the *least squares fit,* is the line that is "best."

This principle will be dealt with a bit further, but it is noted that, just like an average is the number that has the least sum of squares, so is the "best" line defined as the line that has the least "sum of squares" (Figure 10.6). The emphasis on these concepts are made, here, to underline the fact that they are, in a way, axiomatic definitions, and that they are accepted to such a degree that it is possible, at times, that the "best" line is not the least squares fit line, and in modeling, in particular, this *can* be the case.

The line that applies to the data in Table 10.1 is shown in Figure 10.6. It

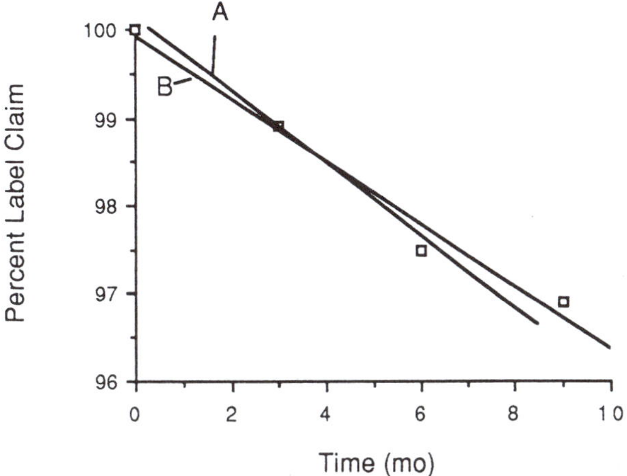

Figure 10.5 Two choices of lines that "run through" the points in Figure 10.4.

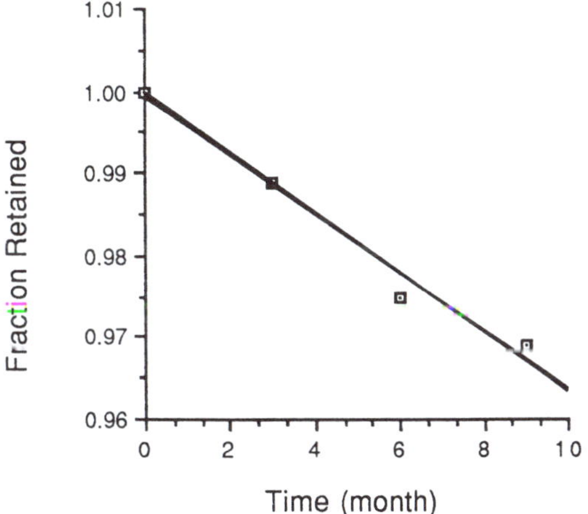

Figure 10.6 The best fit of the "real" line in Figure 10.4, the one with the least squares fit line, i.e., where sum of the squares of the distances $(y_i - {}^{\wedge}y)^2$ are at a minimum. ${}^{\wedge}y$ are the points on the line (i.e., the points calculated from the least squares fit equation), and y_i are the experimental points. Theoretical and least squares fit lines from the second and third column of Table 10.1. Least squares fit is $y = 0.99930 - 0.0035667x$ ($R^2 = 0.979$).

is noted that the slopes and intercepts are comparable, albeit not identical. If, indeed, the line in Figures 10.1 and 10.2 is the "true" line, then it is seen that the least squares fit line is an estimate of the true or population line; in fact, it is difficult to distinguish between the two presentation modes in this case.

10.3 DERIVATION OF THE LEAST SQUARES FIT EQUATION

If we consider the experimental x-values, x_i, and, assuming we knew the "best" line

$$y^{\Lambda} = a + bx \tag{10.5}$$

then we could calculate the y_i^{Λ}-value on the line for each experimental x_i-value. This would, in most cases, differ from the experimental y_i-value, and the difference between the two can now be squared and added to the rest of the deviations squared from the line; i.e., the "sum of the squares," SS, is given by

$$\mathrm{SS} = \Sigma(y_i^{\Lambda} - y_i)^2 = \Sigma(a + bx_i - y_i)^2 \tag{10.6}$$

where a and b are the least squares fit parameters we seek. Since SS should be at a minimum, its derivatives with respect to a and b (not x) must equal zero, i.e.,

$$\partial\mathrm{SS}/\partial a = -2\Sigma(a + bx_i - y_i) = 0 \tag{10.7}$$

and

$$\partial\mathrm{SS}/\partial b = -2\Sigma(a + bx_i - y_i)x_i = 0 \tag{10.8}$$

It is noted that $\Sigma a = na,$ where n is the number of determinations, so these equations rearrange to

$$na + (\Sigma x_i)b = \Sigma y_i \tag{10.9}$$

and

$$(\Sigma x_i)a + (\Sigma x_i^2)b = (\Sigma x_i y_i) \tag{10.10}$$

Employing the determinant approach to solving simultaneous equations now gives

$$\text{Slope} = b = \{n(\Sigma x_i y_i) - (\Sigma x_i \Sigma y_i)\}/\{n(\Sigma x_i^2) - [\Sigma x_i^2]\} \quad (10.11)$$

and

$$\text{Intercept} = a = [(\Sigma y_i) - (b\Sigma x_i)]/n \quad (10.12)$$

10.4 A LONG-HAND EXAMPLE

Suppose that we "knew" that the decay of a drug substance in a given environment (dosage form) was given by

$$y_{\text{theory}} = 100 - 0.003x \quad (10.13)$$

This is not an unrealistic rate constant (b) if it were drawn from room temperature stability data. In reality, there is, however, a certain "error" associated with each "number," e.g., assay error and content uniformity to mention two. The real data would, therefore, be more likely to appear as the third column in Table 10.1 and in Figure 10.7.

The least squares fit of the data in Table 10.1 (expressed in fraction rather than in percentage), when calculated from the previous equations, is given by

$$y^{\wedge} = 0.99930 - 0.0035667x \quad (10.14)$$

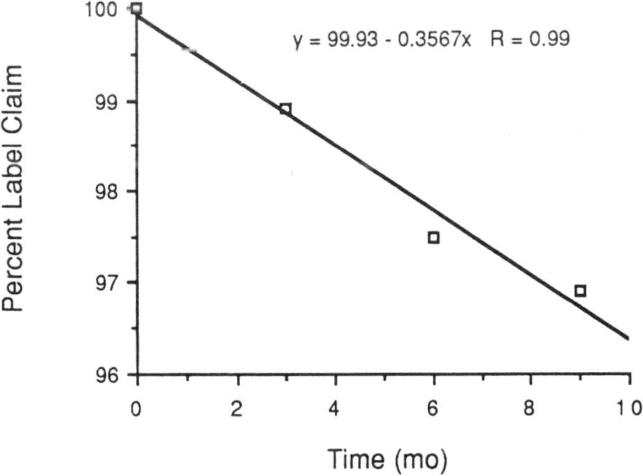

Figure 10.7 Least squares fit line of the data in Table 10.1.

It is noted that this is "close" to the theoretical, and it is also noted that, as explained in an earlier chapter, one is estimating the population parameters (the theoretical line) by the least squares fit parameters.

The equivalent to the variance in number sets is, in the case of lines, the sum of squares about the line divided by $n - 2$, the degrees of freedom:

$$s_{yx}^2 = \mathrm{SS}/(n - 2) \tag{10.15}$$

The manner in which this is calculated, *manually,* is shown in Table 10.2, from which it is seen that

$$s_{yx}^2 = 0.000010743/(4 - 2) = 0.0000053715 \tag{10.16}$$

i.e.,

$$s_{yx} = 0.0023 \tag{10.17}$$

Another quantity that will be needed shortly is

$$\{\Sigma(x - x_{\mathrm{avg}})^2\} = 45^{1/2} = 6.71 \tag{10.18}$$

10.5 THE SLOPE

Frequently, it is the slope that is of importance (e.g., the rate constant), and it is important to be able to assess the precision of this figure. The $100(1 - \beta)\%$ confidence limits (cf) about the slope are given by

$$\mathrm{cf}_{(1-\beta)} = \pm\ t_{n-2,\beta} s_{yx}/\{\Sigma(x - x_{\mathrm{avg}})^2\} \tag{10.19}$$

In the example in Table 10.2, this quantity (for $\beta = 0.05$) would be

$$\mathrm{cf} = 4.303 \cdot 0.0023/6.71 = 0.0015$$

TABLE 10.2. Manual Sum of Squares Calculation.

Time	y	y^	10^4(y-y^)	10^6(y-y^)^2
0	1	0.99930	7	0.49
3	0.989	0.9886	4	0.16
6	0.975	0.9779	29	8.41
9	0.969	0.96772	12.8	1.683
Sum of Squares, SS				10.743

To reiterate, there are two degrees of freedom, and t for 2 df is 4.303 at $\beta = 0.95$. It is noted that the 95% confidence limits for the slope are

$$b = 0.003567 \pm 0.0015 \tag{10.20}$$

It is noted that the limits are wide for several reasons:

(1) the number of determination is small, so t is large.

(2) the length of the x-interval is small, making $\{\Sigma(x - x_{avg})^2\}$ small.

(3) The scatter is moderate to large, so that s_{yx} is large.

It is noted that the meaning of the 95% confidence interval is that one states with 95% confidence that the slope of the population is within the given interval.

10.6 THE INTERCEPT AND EXTRAPOLATED ESTIMATIONS

Given the equation

$$y^{\wedge} = a + bx \tag{10.21}$$

it is, of course, possible to estimate the "best" value of $y_i^{\wedge}$ for any value of x_i. For instance, one may easily calculate that the estimated value for $y^{\wedge}$ at $x = 12$ is

$$y_{12}^{\wedge} = 0.9993 - 0.0035667 \cdot 12 = 0.9565 \tag{10.22}$$

But the question is how good that value is. Again, it can be shown with $100 - \beta\%$ confidence that an interval about the predicted value, x_i, is given by

$$\text{cf} = t_{n-2,\beta} s_{yx}[(1/n) + \{(x_i - x_{avg})^2/\Sigma(x - x_{avg})^2\}]^{1/2} \tag{10.23}$$

It predicts with $(100 - \beta)\%$ confidence that the population line will pass through that interval. Traces of $x_i \pm$ cf are denoted *upper and lower confidence bounds*. For instance, at $x_i = 12$ months, $x_{avg} = 4.5$ so

$$(x_i - x_{avg})^2 = (12 - 4.5)^2 = 56.25 \tag{10.24}$$

From Table 10.2, it is seen that $\Sigma(x - x_{avg})^2 = 45$, and inserting $x_i = 12$ and $s_{yx} = 0.0023$ then gives the term under the square root sign as

$$(1/n) + \{(x_i - x_{avg})^2/\Sigma(x - x_{avg})^2\} = 0.25 + ((12 - 4.5)^2/45) = 1.5 \tag{10.25}$$

so the 90% two-sided interval ($t^{(2)}_{2,0.90} = 2.92$) is given by

$$y = 0.9565 \pm \{2.92 \times 0.0023 \times (1.5^{1/2})\} = 0.957 \pm 0.008 \tag{10.26}$$

It should be noted that what this confidence interval means is the following: there is 90% confidence that the population average will be in this interval for the given value of x_i. Equally well, there is a 95% confidence that the average line will lie above 0.957 − 0.008 = 0.949 = 0.95.

10.7 PREDICTION INTERVALS

If it is desired to calculate the confidence interval in which a specific value will lie, denoting the prediction limit or the upper and lower prediction bounds, the formula is

$$t_{n-2,\beta}s_{yx}[((N + 1)/N) + \{(x_i - x_{avg})^2/\Sigma(x - x_{avg})^2\}]^{1/2} \tag{10.27}$$

In the example above, this would amount to

$$\text{cf} = 2.92 \times 0.0023 \times [1.25 + (56.25/45)]^{1/2}$$

$$= 2.92 \times 0.0023 \times 1.58 = 0.016 \tag{10.28}$$

This then predicts the 90% confidence (probability) that the true values of the population at that point in time will lie in the calculated interval or that, with 95% confidence, the values will be above 0.957 − 0.016 = 0.941 = 0.94.

10.8 THE CORRELATION COEFFICIENT, *R*

The coefficient of determination, denoted R^2, is given by

$$R^2 = b^2[\Sigma(x - x_{avg})^2]/[\Sigma(y - y_{avg})^2]$$

$$= [\Sigma(xy) - \{\Sigma(x)\Sigma(y)/n\}]^2/[\Sigma(x - x_{avg})^2][\Sigma(y - y_{avg})^2] \tag{10.29}$$

and its square root, R, is denoted the correlation coefficient.

The correlation coefficient essentially states that "when x goes up, y goes up" ($R = +1$) or "when x goes down, y goes up" ($R = -1$).

It can be shown in this set of data (Table 10.1) that the correlation coefficient is

$$R = -0.989 \tag{10.30}$$

The correlation coefficient is given with nines until a non-nine appears, e.g., in the above case, $R = 0.99$ would be the best presentation mode.

Often, the statement is made that the "data fit well" because the correlation coefficient is close to plus or minus one. But how close does it have to be to be "significant"?

It can be shown that the quantity

$$Q = R[(n - 2)/(1 - R^2)]^{1/2} \tag{10.31}$$

is distributed by student-t with $n - 2$ degrees of freedom. In the above case,

$$Q = 0.989[2/(1 - 0.978)]^{1/2} = 0.989[2/0.022]^{1/2} = 9.4 > 4.3$$

and since this exceeds $t_{2,0.05} = 4.3$, we reject the null hypotheses and show that there, indeed, is a correlation.

With few data points, investigators will often cite that the fit is good if the correlation coefficient is, e.g., 0.9. Had this been the case above, then

$$Q = 0.9[2/(1 - 0.81)]^{1/2} = 1.9$$

i.e., a correlation coefficient of 0.9 would not suffice to "guarantee" a correlation. Conversely, if a large number of data points (e.g., $n = 1000$) is on hand, then relatively small correlation coefficients (e.g., 0.7) suffice to "guarantee" a correlation.

10.9 UPPER AND LOWER CONFIDENCE BOUNDS: PROGRAMMING THE LEAST SQUARES FIT

In many situations (e.g., in expiration period calculations), it is convenient to show the upper and lower 95% or 90% confidence bounds or prediction bounds. It is seen above how the 95% (or other confidence) limits can be calculated for any point in time (interpolation or extrapolation). If this is done in a continuous fashion, then two curves result, viz., what is known as the upper and lower bound for the mean.

As an example, the data in Table 10.3 are stability data that are treated

TABLE 10.3. Stability Data for a New Product. Data in the Last Two Columns Were Calculated from Program 10.

Time (Months) x	y	y^	Lower Confidence Bounds (95% One-Sided)
0	100	99.9	98.95
3	98.5	98.91	98.23
6	98.0	97.93	97.37
9	97.6	96.93	96.25
12	95.5	95.34	94.98
18		93.96	92.31
24		91.98	89.58

in this fashion. The actual manner in which the data were obtained, programmatically, will be discussed further at a later point.

The equation for the lower confidence bounds is

$$y = y^{\wedge} - ts_{yx}[(1/n) + \{(x_i - x_{avg})^2/\Sigma(x - x_{avg})^2\}]^{1/2} \qquad (10.32)$$

and is of the shape shown in Figures 10.8 and 10.9.

10.10 EXPIRATION PERIODS

The 1987 FDA Stability Guidelines recommend that expiration periods be calculated by the method discussed in Section 10.9. In general, the label claim limits in the USP are 90–110% of label claim, so that one (in general) must have some assurance that an "assay" be above 90% of label claim at the end of the expiration period. The ruling for the calculation of the expiration period is that one must ascertain with 95% (one-sided) confidence that the average line (the estimate of the population stability line) be above 90% label claim at the end of the expiration period.

One way of visualizing this graphically is by use of SigmaPlot®, which contains a transform for 95% confidence and prediction bounds. It is easily converted to two-sided 90% (one-sided 95%) confidence bounds by changing the Z-value in the transform program from 1.96 to 1.645.

For the "individual" assays (the prediction limits), the 90% confidence limits (the prediction limits) are

$$\pm\gamma = \pm t_{0.9,1}s_{yx}\{\sqrt{(\{N + 1\}/N) + \{[(x - x^*)^2]/\Sigma(x - x_{avg})^2\}} \qquad (10.33)$$

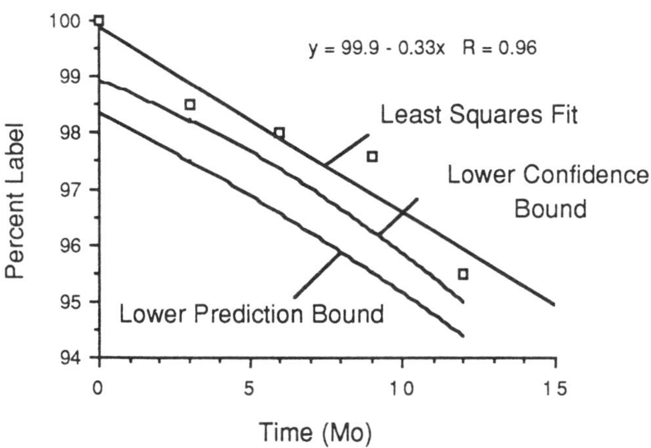

Figure 10.8 Confidence and prediction bounds, as obtained by SigmaPlot®.

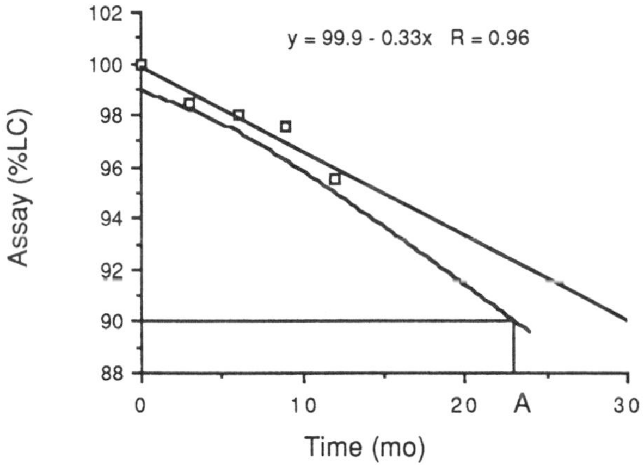

Figure 10.9 Example of expiration period calculation. The lower line is the lower confidence bound calculated in Table 10.3.

This is best illustrated by example. Given the stability data in Table 10.3 from a new product, one might ask what the expiration period would be.

The data are calculated according to the formula above, and the data are graphed in Figure 10.9. It is seen that the calculated expiration period would be about 24 months.

10.11 PROGRAMS FOR REGRESSION WITH CONFIDENCE BOUNDS

Rather than calculating least squares fits and confidence bounds by hand, programs can be written to carry out the calculations.

10.11.1 PROGRAM IN BASIC

The program in Table 10.4 is a BASIC program.

The parameter values obtained are identical to those in Figure 10.9. The data are input in the 400-bank, and if the program is to be used for other data sets, these should be entered in this bank. Note that the data can be entered in one line as well, i.e.,

```
400 DATA 0.100,3,98.5,6,98,9,97.6,12,95.5
```

The program contains actual t-values and the approximation function for t (90% two-sided, 95% one-sided) derived in Appendix 4 at the end of the book has been used for $N2 > 9$.

When the program is executed, it asks for the number, N, of determinations, and once this is inserted, it will print out:

(1) A table of x- and y-values
(2) The slope, intercept, and correlation coefficient
(3) The lower confidence bound and the upper and lower prediction bounds after the time periods indicated in step 965

For ordinary stability programs this would be

```
965 FOR J2 = 0 to 60 STEP 6
```

The printed output is obtained by placing an L before all the PRINT statements in the program in some configurations.

The situation often arises where two sets of data are fairly close, and it is desirable to see whether the slopes differ and whether the data can be pooled as if from a common population [Snedocor and Cochran (1982)].

TABLE 10.4. Program for Calculating the Regression Line and Confidence Bounds (95% One-Sided, 90% Two-Sided).

```
100 PRINT "Expiration Period Program"
110 INPUT "NO OF POINTS="; N1
120 PRINT "No of Points=";N1
150 PRINT "TIME", "CONCENTRATION"
160  PRINT  "------------------------"
170 N2 = 0
200 READ A,B
210 N2 = N2 + 1
220 X = A
230 Y =B
240 X1 = X1+X
250 X2 = X2 + (X^2)
260 Y1 = Y1 +Y
270 Y2 = Y2 + (Y^2)
280 Z1 =Z1 + (X*Y)
300 PRINT X,Y
310 IF N2 = N1 GOTO 700
320 GOTO 200
350 REM "DATA IS INPUTTED AS A,B"
401 DATA 0, 100
402 DATA 3, 98.5
403 DATA 6, 98
404 DATA 9,97.6
405 DATA 12,95.5
700 Z2 = x2-(x1^2/N2)
710 Z3 = Y2 - (Y1^2/N2)
720 Z4 = Z1 -(X1*Y1/N2)
730 Z5 = Z4/Z2
800  PRINT  "----------------------------"
800 PRINT "SLOPE= ";Z5
810 Z6 = (Y1-(Z5* X1))/N2
820 PRINT "INTERCEPT= ";Z6
830 Z7 = (Z4^2)/(Z3*Z2)
840 Z8 = (Z7)^(.5)
860 Z9 - (Z3-(( Z5^2)*Z2))/(N2-2)
973 PRINT "CORREL. COEFF= ";Z8
874 J1 = X1/N2
875 PRINT "time","y^","Low Conf","Low Pred", "Up Pred
880 PRINT  "                    Bd Avg"  ,"Bd Indiv.", "Bd
                                                          Indiv
888 IF N2 = 3 THEN T = 6.3138
889 IF N2 = 4 THEN T = 2.9200
890 IF N2 = 5 THEN T = 2.3534
891 IF N2 = 6 THEN T = 2.1318
892 IF N2 = 7 THEN T = 2.0150
893 IF N2 = 8 THEN T = 1.9432
894 IF N2 = 9 THEN T = 1.8946
895 IF N2 >9 THEN T = 1.645 + (1/(-0.556 + (.6555*N2)))
965 FOR J2 = 0 TO 24 STEP 4
```

(continued)

TABLE 10.4. *(continued).*

```
970 J3 = Z6 + (Z5*J2)
972 J7 = (1/N2) + (((J2-J1)^2)/Z2)
975 J8 = J7^.5
980 J9 = T*(Z9^(.5))*J8
985 D4 = J3 - J9
990 D5 = ((N2+1)/N2) + (((J2-J1)^2)/Z2)
991 G1 = D5^(.5)
992 G2 = T*(Z9^(.5))*G1
985 D6 = J3 - G2
986 D7 = J3 + G2
987 PRINT J2, J3, D4, D6, D7
1000 NEXT J2
1960 U1 = Z6 + (Z5*X)
 970 U2 = (1/N2) + (((X-J1)^2)/Z2)
 975 U3 = U2^.5
 980 U4 = T*(Z9^(.5))*U3
 985 U5 = U1 - U4
 987 PRINT "Low Conf Bd Avg=";U5
 990 U6 = ((N2+1)/N2) + (((X-J1)^2)/Z2)
 991 U7 = U6^(.5)
 992 U8 = T*(Z9^(.5))*U7
 985 U9 = U1 - U8
 986 K1 = U1+U8
 987 PRINT "Low Pred Bd Ind=";U9
 988 PRINT "Up Pred Bd Ind=";K1
 2000 END
```

One criterion for this is that $[\{SS - (SS_1^2 + SS_2^2)\}/2]/\{(SS_1^2 + SS_2^2)/(n_1 + n_2 - 4)\} < F_{crit}(2, n_1 + n_2 - 4)$. A program is available through the FDA for carrying out this test.

If the number of determinations, N, is increased, then the confidence intervals will become narrower. In stability programs (and other experimental situations), there are usually several batches, and if they are combined in the estimate, N, of course, will increase. On the other hand, s_{yx} will increase, and in the limit, adverse effects may result. This (somewhat unusual case) is demonstrated in Figure 10.10.

If assays could be normalized (e.g., to percent or fraction of label claim), then the above would pose no problem. The FDA stability guidelines, however, specifically prohibit such an approach.

10.11.2 SIGMAPLOT®

An excellent program for many situations is SigmaPlot®. This program has the advantage of showing, in its manuals, the transform programs and, for instance, lists a Regression with Confidence Transform. The confidence limits are 95% (Z = 1.96), but this is easily corrected to 90% by simply changing to Z = 1.645 should that be desired, as it is in the program below.

The method is simply the following (for Macintosh):

(1) The SigmaPlot® application is double-clicked.
(2) The data are entered in the first two columns of the worksheet, i.e.,
  - Column 1 contains the "real" time values.
  - Column 2 contains the "real" *y*-values.
(3) Under the math heading, TRANSFORM is selected (blacked out). Click NEW and select the Regression Program from the menu.
(4) Click OK. (The program now runs.)
(5) A series of columns will appear:
  - Column 3 contains *x*-values for the plotting of the confidence limits.
  - Column 4 contains the $y^{\wedge}$ values.
  - Column 5 contains the upper confidence bound values.
  - Column 6 contains the lower confidence bound values.
  - Column 7 contains the upper prediction bound values.
  - Column 8 contains the lower prediction bound values.

In plotting, the problem is that there are two *x*-columns. This is best handled as follows.

(6) Under FILE, drag to DEFAULT and then one column over to CANCEL (Default→Cancel).
(7) Click/drag GRAPH→CARTESIAN.

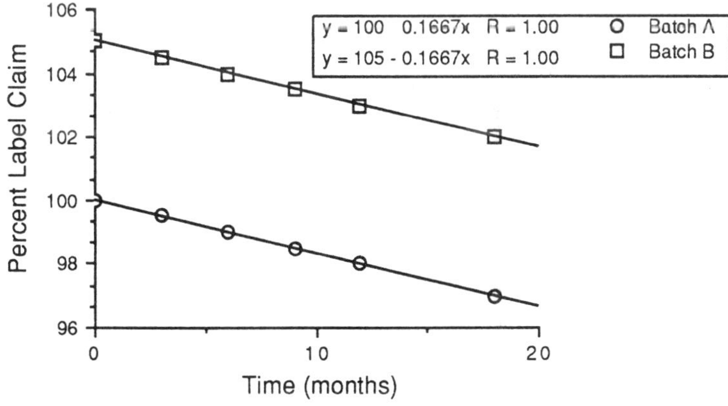

Figure 10.10 A case where pooling is not advantageous.

(8) Leave on PAIRWISE *x,y*. Click WORKSHEET. The program asks for what column to consider *x*.
(9) Click Column 1. The program asks for what column to consider *y*.
(10) Click Column 2.
(11) Click DONE.
(12) Click/drag DRAW GRAPH→CARTESIAN again.
(13) Click the T VERSUS ROW SELECTION, then click WORKSHEET.
(14) The program asks for what column to consider *y*.
(15) Click columns 4, 5, 6, 7, and 8.
(16) Click DONE.
(17) A graph will appear with (a) the points, (b) the least squares fit, (c) the upper and lower confidence bounds, and (d) the upper and lower prediction limits.

10.11.3 STATWORKS™

It was mentioned in Chapter 3 that StatWorks™ is used in this book. When used for regression, there are a series of outputs. The first output is simply the data (this StatWorks™ output is not shown), and the second is a graph of the data (not shown either). There then follow two tables. The first gives a *t*-test evaluation of the data, and shows that

(1) The data fail to show a difference of the intercept from 1.00 (first line, entry: "Constant").
(2) There is a 98.9% (1–0.011) probability that the regression is real.

The second table is an ANOVA table, showing, again, that there is a 98.9% probability of the regression being real. It gives the correlation coefficient (the "adjustment" is outside the scope of this text and can be disregarded for this purpose).

What is denoted the "standard error of the estimate" is s_{yx}.

10.12 ASSUMPTIONS MADE IN THE LEAST SQUARES FIT

The least squares fit is employed in many situations. There are several assumptions that are made in this computation, and these are often not recognized or are simply ignored. The most salient assumptions are

(1) The *x*-values are precise.
(2) The *y*-values are normally distributed.
(3) There is no curvature.

TABLE 10.5. Sample Stability Data.

Time	Assay
0	100
4	98
8	90
12	82
Average	92.5

Of these, x is often the case. If a kinetic study is carried out, for instance, the recording of time is much more precise than the assay of the sample, so that, most often, the condition (1) is adhered to.

The second condition, (2) is taken for granted, but, particularly when data are transformed, this is not realistic. An example of this will be given later. The last assumption is one that is also often overlooked, and this will be treated as well. An example of this will be given later.

10.13 ANOVA OF LEAST SQUARES FIT

Most programs, e.g., StatWorks™, will analyze the data by way of ANOVA. An example would be, again, a set of stability data, the data in Table 10.5.

The question arises whether there is a "trend," i.e., whether the assay is dropping with time. To this end, the (regression) line (y_c) and the (experimental) points (y_i) are compared with the "average" line (the horizontal line in Figure 10.11, i.e., y_{avg} = 92.5%). If there were no trend, then the

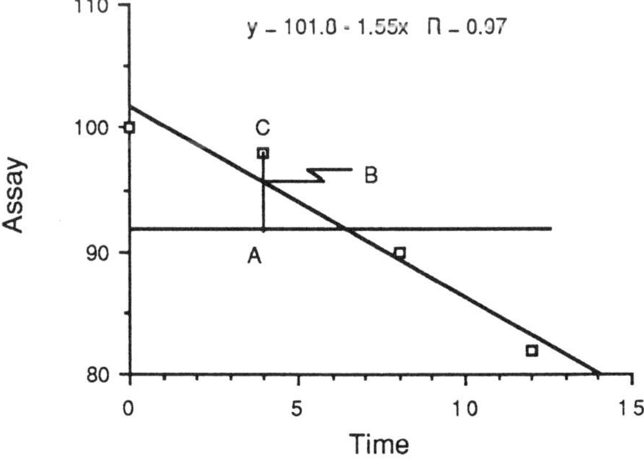

Figure 10.11 Schematic for discussion of ANOVA for regression lines.

two "should be the same." As an example (the second point), the distance *AB* is the "explained" deviation ($y_c - y_i$) from the average to the line, and *CB* is the "unexplained" deviation. The "total" deviation ($y_i - y_{avg}$) is *AC*.
It follows that

$$(y_i - y_{avg}) = (y_c - y_{avg}) + (y_i - y_c) \tag{10.34}$$

It is now conventional to state that

$$\Sigma(y_i - y_{avg})^2 = \Sigma(y_c - y_{avg})^2 + \Sigma(y_i - y_c)^2 \tag{10.35}$$

which is correct, mathematically, if

$$\Sigma 2(y_c - y_{avg})(y_i - y_c) = 0 \tag{10.36}$$

Denoting by "SS" the sum of squares, the terms in Equation (10.35) are

$$\Sigma(y_i - y_{avg})^2 = SS_{total} \tag{10.37}$$

$$\Sigma(y_c - y_{avg})^2 = SS_{explained} \tag{10.38}$$

$$\Sigma(y_i - y_c)^2 = SS_{unexplained} \tag{10.39}$$

The total sum of squares, SS_{total}, is a measure of how much the observed *y*-values are dispersed about their mean value, y_{avg}. The explained sum of squares, $SS_{explained}$, is a measure of whatever variability in the observed *y*-values is accounted for by the linear relationship, and the unexplained sum of squares, or as it is also called, the residual sum of squares, $SS_{unexplained}$, is a measure of how much the observed *Y*-values are scattered about the least squares fit line. It is $SS_{unexplained}$ that is minimized to obtain the equation for the least squares fit line.

The parameter that determines whether there is a positive correlation between *x* and *y* is the ANOVA ratio:

$$RV = SS_{explained}/SS_{residual} \tag{10.40}$$

On the other hand, the correlation coefficient, *R* (coefficient of determination, R^2), is given by

$$R^2 = SS_{explained}/SS_{total} \tag{10.41}$$

A StatWorks™ program of the data in Table 10.5 is shown in Table 10.6. The standard error of estimate, 2.324, is the residual sum of squares

TABLE 10.6. Analysis of Data from Table 10.5 by StatWorks™.

Data File: Table 10.5

Source	Sum of Squares	Deg. of Freedom	Mean Squares	F-Ratio	Prob>F
Model	192.200000	1	192.200000	35.592593	0.027
Error	10.800000	2	5.400000		
Total	203.000000	3			

Coefficient of Determination (R^2)	0.946798
Adjusted Coefficient (R^2)	0.920197
Coefficient of Correlation (R)	0.973035
Standard Error of Estimate	2.323790
Durbin-Watson Statistic	3.190476

divided by $N - 2$. The Durbin-Watson Statistic will be discussed in a later section. The coefficient of determination, 0.947, is seen to be according to Equation (10.41), in that

$$192/203 = 0.946$$

10.14 WEIGHTED LEAST SQUARES

It happens that each point may not carry the same "weight" as other points. An example of this is shown in Table 10.7 where the effect of a ligand on the rate constant of a drug substance is studied. The two species, A and B, will complex, and the decomposition reaction will occur from both the drug A and the complex {AB}, but at different rates.

Suppose the variance (standard error of the estimate squared) of the determined rate constants are as shown. We would then want to "count"

TABLE 10.7. Example of Weighting.

	Concentration of Ligand	Rate Constant	Variance	f	w (f/19.5)
A	0.1	0.01	0.001	10	0.513
B	0.2	0.0155	0.005	2	0.103
C	0.3	0.021	0.002	5	0.256
D	0.4	0.024	0.004	2.5	0.128
Totals				19.5	1.00

A five times as much as B and C, 2.5 times as much as A, and so on. One may do this as shown in the last column (w). The number of points of A is then $4 \cdot 0.513 = 2.052$, the number of points of B is $4 \cdot 0.103 = 0.412$, and so on.

10.15 SIGNIFICANCE OF CORRELATION AND CURVATURE

So far, all data have been treated as if they were linear. Many situations are linear or pseudolinear (pseudo-zero-order) in nature, but most often, this manifestation is simply approximate. One example of this has been mentioned, viz., that a first-order reaction will appear linear (when assay variances are in the "normal" pharmaceutical range) when the decomposition is less than 15%.

10.16 THE SIGNIFICANCE OF THE CORRELATION COEFFICIENT

Whenever a statement is made, it is associated with a level of confidence, yet most all investigators use the correlation coefficient with statements such as "good correlation because the correlation coefficient is close to 1.0."

Even worse, as shall be seen below, many authors state that "there is good linearity as witnessed by the fact that the correlation coefficient is close to unity." This author himself can be accused of that occasionally.

Given a set of data as shown in Table 10.7, one obviously obtains a

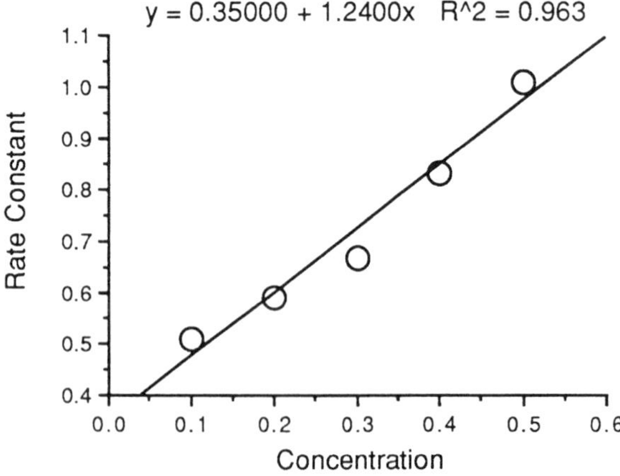

Figure 10.12 Data from Table 10.8.

TABLE 10.8. Rate Constants as a Function of Drug Concentration.

Concentration (mM)	0.1	0.2	0.3	0.4	0.5
Rate Constant (hr^{-1})	0.51	0.59	0.67	0.83	1.01

"good" correlation coefficient. As mentioned earlier, this need not imply correlation, because the number depends on the number of determinations in the set.

If one inspects the data in Figure 10.12 (and Table 10.8), it is obvious, from visual examination, that there is an S-type trend in the plot, but the correlation coefficient is still quite good. The data output on StatWorks™ is shown in Table 10.9. The standard error of the estimate in this table is the value of s, and the Durbin-Watson statistic will be touched on below.

As mentioned, correlation coefficients are a function of the number of determinations. It is also noted that the StatWorks™-output shows the ANOVA F-ratio and gives the probability of that F being superseded, i.e., in this case, quite small (0.3%). Again, this does not imply linearity, simply correlation. Curvature is addressed in the last line of tabular StatWorks™ outputs (e.g., Table 10.9) in terms of the Durbin-Watson statistic.

10.17 DURBIN-WATSON STATISTICS

Durbin-Watson (DW) statistics probe the possibility of curvature by the

TABLE 10.9. Linear Output from the Data in Table 10.8 Using StatWorks™.

Data File: Table 10.5 Dependent Variable: Rate Constant

Variable Name	Coefficient	Std. Err. Estimate	t Statistic	Prob > t
Constant	0.354000	0.039056	9.064020	0.003
Drug Conc.	1.240000	0.117757	10.530176	0.002

Data File: Table 10.5

Source	Sum of Squares	Deg. of Freedom	Mean Squares	F-Ratio	Prob>F
Model	0.153760	1	0.153760	110.884615	0.002
Error	0.004160	3	0.001387		
Total	0.157920	4			

Coefficient of Determination (R^2)	0.973658
Adjusted Coefficient (R^2)	0.964877
Coefficient of Correlation (R)	0.986741
Standard Error of Estimate	0.037238
Durbin-Watson Statistic	1.882653

following procedure. If the quantity

$$y_i - y^{\wedge} = e_i \tag{10.42}$$

is calculated for each point, then one may calculate the statistic, DW, given by

$$\mathrm{DW} = \sum_{i=2}^{i=n} (e_j - e_{j-1})^2 / \Sigma e_i^2 \tag{10.43}$$

If there is no "autocorrelation," this term should be zero (H_0: DW $= 0$), and hence one postulates by null hypothesis that it is, and calculates the likelihood of this. Upper (d_u) and lower (d_l) limits for DW have been published (for $n > 15$), and the criteria are that

$$\mathrm{DW} > d_u: \quad H_0 \text{ is concluded (no curvature)} \tag{10.44}$$

$$\mathrm{DW} < d_l: \quad H_1 \text{ is concluded (curvature)} \tag{10.45}$$

$$d_u > \mathrm{DW} > d_l: \quad \text{test is inconclusive} \tag{10.46}$$

It is noted that the StatWorks™ output gives the Durbin-Watson statistics without implying a level of significance. The values for d_l and d_u are shown in Figure 10.13, but are not really reliable below $N = 15$.

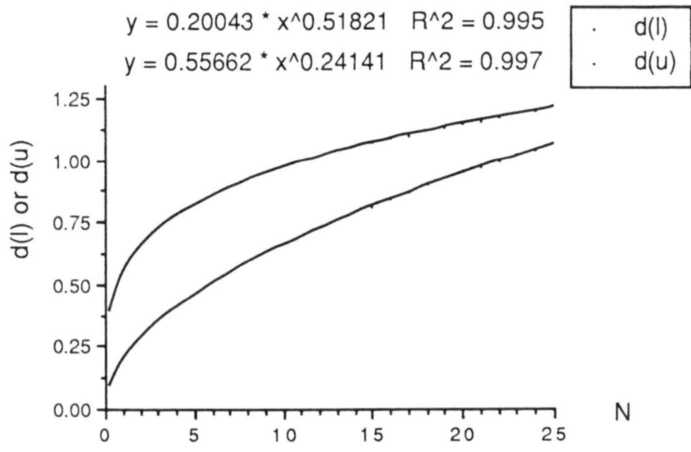

Figure 10.13 Durbin-Watson limits at the $\alpha = 0.01$ level.

TABLE 10.10. Durbin-Watson limits at the $\alpha = 0.01$ level.

Concentration (mM)	0.1	0.2	0.3	0.4	0.5
Rate Constant (hr^{-1})	0.51	0.59	0.67	0.83	1.01
Second variable, x_2.	0.01	0.04	0.09	0.16	0.25

10.18 MULTIPLE REGRESSION

When a property (y) is a function of several variables, then the principle of least squares can be used in the same fashion as when only two variables are involved. For two independent variables (x_1 and x_2), there will be three differential equations. The solution to these (a, b, and c) will be of the form:

$$y = a + bx_1 + cx_2 \tag{10.47}$$

Given the set of data in Table 10.10, multiple regression can be performed and is done so in Table 10.11.

In using StatWorks™, the selection multiple regression is sought out (under regression), and the dependent variables are the two last lines, and the concentration is the independent variable. The output is shown in Table 10.11.

TABLE 10.11. Data from Table 10.10 Treated by StatWorks™ Multiple Regression.

Data File: Table 10.9 — Dependent Variable: Rate Constant

Variable Name	Coefficient	Std. Err. Estimate	t Statistic	Prob > t
Constant	0.474000	0.010254	46.226227	0.000
Drug Conc.	0.211429	0.078142	2.705708	0.073
Salt Conc.	1.714286	0.127775	13.416408	0.001

Data File: Table 10.9

Source	Sum of Squares	Deg. of Freedom	Mean Squares	F-Ratio	Prob>F
Model	0.157874	2	0.078937	3453.500000	0.000
Error	0.000046	2	0.000023		
Total	0.157920	4			

Coefficient of Determination (R^2)	0.999711
Adjusted Coefficient (R^2)	0.999421
Coefficient of Correlation (R)	0.999855
Standard Error of Estimate	0.004781
Durbin-Watson Statistic	3.072581

TABLE 10.12. Logarithmic Decay Data.

Time	y_{th} ($e^{-=0.4x}$)	y_{exp}	ln[y_{exp}]
0	0	1	0
1	0.67	0.84	-0.174
2	0.449	0.279	-1.277
3	0.301	0.386	-0.952
4	0.202	0.117	-2.146
5	0.135	0.170	-1.772
6	0.091	0.056	-2.882

10.19 TRANSFORMATIONS

In treating transformed variables, there is a problem when utilizing least squares regression, because if, for instance, y is normally distributed, then ln [y] is *not* normally distributed, and in general, if y is normally distributed, then the transformed variable is not.

In most cases, this does not much matter, but in some cases, it does. One case where it is not too serious is in logarithmic transformations. Take, for instance, the data in Table 10.12. These data are obtained from the theoretical curve

$$y = e^{-0.4x} \tag{10.48}$$

Errors are placed on the theoretical points to obtain the "experimental" points, and the third column in Table 10.12 results, and these results are shown in Figure 10.14.

If we traditionally took logarithms of the fraction retained and did least squares fit on this, then the least squares fit line is as shown in Figure 10.15.

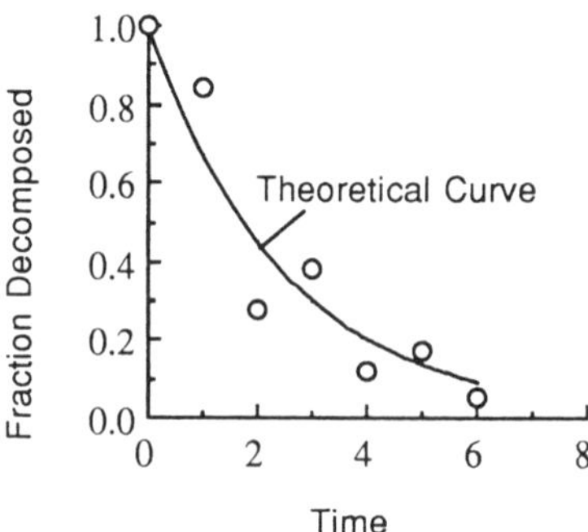

Figure 10.14 Data from Table 10.12.

More significant figures are carried in this case, so that the exponentialization later will not suffer.

$$\ln [y] = 0.04726182 - 0.4539805x \qquad (10.49)$$

As noted in Figure 10.15, this is exactly the figure obtained in the CricketGraph™ so the program in CricketGraph™ must have been obtained by the same logarithmic transformation shown in Table 10.2. Here, the least squares fit is obtained by transformation in the last column. To assess how good the fit is, it is first necessary to exponentialize Equation (10.49):

$$y^{\wedge} = \exp(0.047262 + 0.45398x)$$

and then calculate the sum of squares from the (untransformed) y-values:

$$\Sigma(y_{\text{exp}} - y^{\wedge})^2 = 7.4003 \cdot 10^{-1}$$

By testing a couple of other combinations, it is obvious from Table 10.13 that

$$y^{\wedge} = \exp(0.0474 + 0.453x)$$

gives a better fit. The mere fact that one combination can be found that gives a smaller sum of squares shows that least squares fitting of the transformed variable does not give the best fit. However, the estimates by transformation, in the case of logarithmic transformations, are usually quite good.

An even better fit is obtained by SigmaPlot® by fitting the data

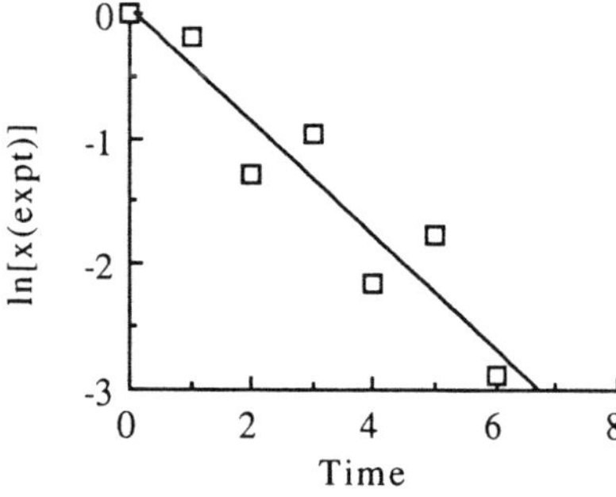

Figure 10.15 Data from the fourth column in Table 10.2. The least squares fit is ln $[y] = 0.047262 - 0.45398x$ ($R^2 = 0.885$).

TABLE 10.13. Sum of Squares of Different Fits of the Experimental Data in Table 10.12.

	Transformed Eq. 10.49	Fit by Eye	SigmaPlot®
Slope[a]	0.0474	0.0473	0.047262
Intercept[a]	0.453	0.454	0.45398
10^2 x Sum of Squares	7.3839	7.4004	7.4003

[a] of the logarithmic transformation, e.g. as shown in Fig. 10.15.

nonlinearly to an equation of the form of Equation (10.48). The result is that the pertinent data from this fitting is shown in Table 10.13.

$$y = 1.047e^{-0.4261}$$

10.20 NONLINEAR REGRESSION

As mentioned, it is possible, by trial and error, to find a fit for which

$$y = e^{-a+bx}$$

is more adequate than the transformed treatment. As in Table 10.13, other values may be tried, and there will be one set of values of a and b, which will give the least sum of squares.

There are programs such as SigmaPlot® that will do just that, but it should be pointed out that they work by an iteration procedure. Here, it is necessary to have initial estimates of the parameters, and for the procedure to be successful, it is necessary to have good estimates, and one way of getting them is to first do transformed plotting and use the parameter values thusly obtained as first estimates in the nonlinear program. This will be the subject of the next chapter.

10.21 WEIGHTING OF TRANSFORMED VARIABLES

There are two ways of overcoming the adverse effects of transformations on least squares fitting. One is by weighting the variables.

The x and y values of two parameters that are reciprocally related are shown in the first two columns of Tables 10.14 and 10.15. Suppose the y-value has a precision of 0.01 absolute units. Then the limits would be as shown in the third and fourth lines of the table.

TABLE 10.14. Reciprocally Related Variables, *x* and *y*.

x	y	ymin	ymax	1/ymin	1/ymax	r	1/r2
2	0.6	0.57	0.63	1.75	1.59	0.16	39.0
1	0.39	0.37	0.41	2.70	2.44	0.26	14.8
0.25	0.14	0.133	0.147	7.69	6.80	0.89	1.26
0.1	0.06	0.057	0.063	17.54	15.87	1.67	0.36
0.04	0.02	0.019	0.021	52.63	47.62	5.01	0.04
						Total	55.46

It is assumed here that the variance on each figure is proportional to the range squared, so that $1/r^2$ is used as a weighting factor, then each point is weighted according to its variance, the one with the largest variance counting the least. Weighting is shown in Table 10.15.

The total number in the calculation must equal five (since manipulations cannot increase the number of degrees of freedom). A weighted least squares can now be carried out. This is done in a fashion similar to that shown for the program for least squares fitting, except that the READ statement is now A,B,C where C is the weighting factor. The following parameter values are found:

$$\text{Slope} = 1.7125 \tag{10.50}$$

$$\text{Intercept} = 0.8063 \tag{10.51}$$

$$\text{Correlation Coefficient} = 0.994 \tag{10.52}$$

10.22 POLYNOMIALS

Often, there will be curvature in data, which may be aproximated by a polynomial. As an example, the data in Table 10.16 show the defects (in 10^{-2} × Percentage) of bottles on a packing line as a function of line speed.

TABLE 10.15. Weighting of Data from Table 10.14 Inversely to the Variance.

x	y	1/r2.	f	N
2	0.6	39.0	0.7032	3.5159
1	0.39	14.8	0.2669	1.3345
0.25	0.14	1.26	0.0227	0.1135
0.1	0.06	0.36	0.0065	0.0325
0.04	0.02	0.04	0.0007	0.0036
		55.46	1.0000	5.0000

TABLE 10.16. Defects as a Function of Line Speed.

Speed x	10^2 x Defect Percent (y)	x^2 (or z)
0	1.8	0
2	3.3	4
4	4	16
6	4.9	36
8	6.7	64
10	7.8	100

The data are plotted in Figure 10.16. It is visually seen that there is curvature, and as a first approximation, a second-order polynomial fit is attempted. The fit seems quite good. The question that might arise is how this fit was accomplished.

If the data are considered as being a set where y is multiple regressed, i.e., if $x^2 = z$, then the polynomial may be written

$$y = a + bx + cz \tag{10.53}$$

and multiple regressing the second column of Table 10.16 against the two other columns should give a, b, and c in

$$y = a + bx + cx^2 \tag{10.54}$$

This is done in Table 10.17.

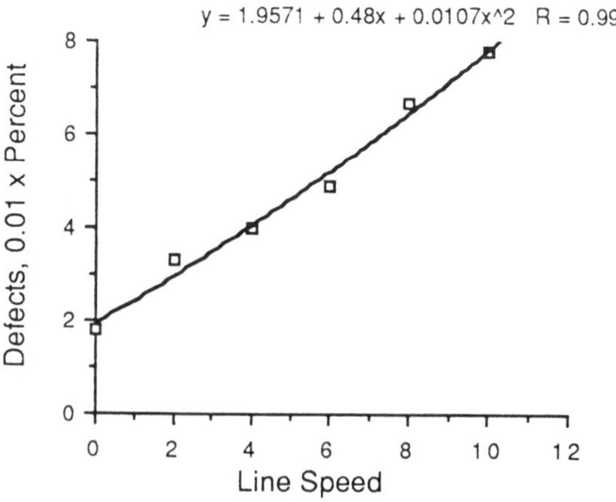

Figure 10.16 Data from Table 10.16.

TABLE 10.17. Multiple Regression of Data in Table 10.16.

Data File: Untitled Data — Dependent Variable: y

Variable Name	Coefficient	Std. Err. Estimate	t Statistic	Prob > t
Constant	1.957143	0.284139	6.887989	0.002
x	0.480000	0.133634	3.591888	0.023
x squared	0.010714	0.012827	0.835269	0.451

Data File: Untitled Data

Source	Sum of Squares	Deg. of Freedom	Mean Squares	F-Ratio	Prob>F
Model	24.200143	2	12.100071	123.111192	0.001
Error	0.294857	3	0.098286		
Total	24.495000	5			

Coefficient of Determination (R^2)	0.987963
Adjusted Coefficient (R^2)	0.979938
Coefficient of Correlation (R)	0.993963
Standard Error of Estimate	0.313506
Durbin-Watson Statistic	3.054993

It is noted that the coefficients are exactly the same as obtained in Figure 10.16. Whether CricketGraph™ accomplishes polynomial fits by means of multiple regression or whether, in the case of the data at hand, multiple regression of x and z actually gives the same results as nonlinear fitting is difficult to judge. In the latter case, however, the multiple regression treatment would cause a dependency of the coefficients. It should be pointed out that, for most applications, the CricketGraph™ approach is quite adequate.

10.23 LEAST SQUARES FITS OF DISTRIBUTION FUNCTIONS

It happens, in some fields, that data will have the appearance of a distribution function. Dehydration of crystalline hydrates is such an instance, and often, as they dehydrate, they will lose their crystallinity and become amorphous anhydrates. These have a residual amount of moisture, depending on the pressure at which the dehydration took place. A set of such data is shown in Table 10.18.

The data are shown graphically in Figure 10.17. If the profile is thought probabilistic in nature, then it should be a cumulative Gaussian type. Such data could, therefore, be plotted on probability paper, but how does one, in a formal sense, obtain a least squares fit? Also, how does one account for the fact that there is residual moisture in the amorphous "anhydrate"?

TABLE 10.18. Dehydration of a Crystalline Hydrate into an Amorphous Anhydrate.

Time (Min)	% Hydrate (D)	(D-10)/100 =Q	Q/0.9	Z
0	100	0.9	1.0	
2	99	0.89	0.989	2.3
4	95	0.85	0.944	1.6
6	83	0.73	0.811	0.9
8	60	0.50	0.556	0.13
10	30	0.20	0.222	-0.76
12	20	0.10	0.111	-1.21
14	15	0.05	0.056	-1.60
16	10	0	0	

It would appear that the data would level off at some point about ten. This is then subtracted from the figures in column 2 and expressed as fraction crystalline anhydrate, and this is shown in column 3. This is normalized (by division by 0.9, to make the highest "fraction" = 1.0) and is shown in column 4. This corresponds to the "area" figures in a normal error table (if indeed the function is probital in nature), and the corresponding Z-values are found from Appendix 1.

The Z-values are shown in column 5 and are plotted versus time in Figure 10.18. The average x-value is found by setting $Z = 0$, i.e.,

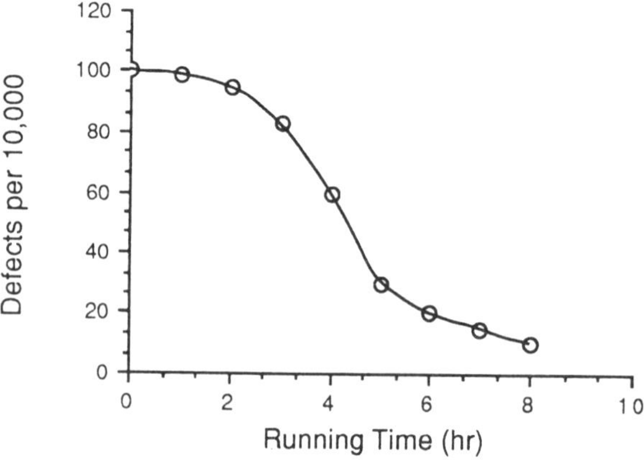

Figure 10.17 Data from Table 10.18.

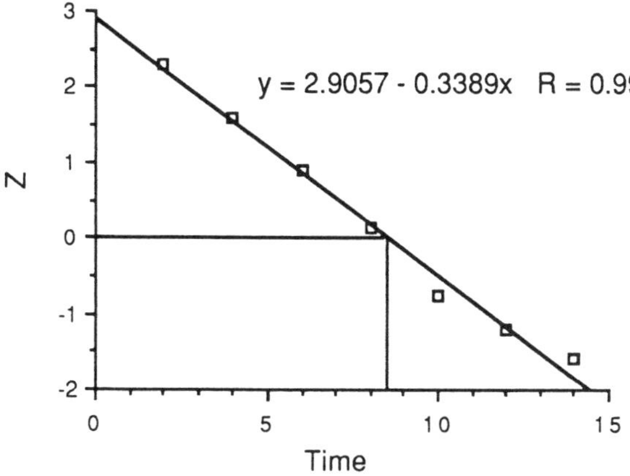

Figure 10.18 Data from Table 10.18 plotted according to a probit function.

$$x_{avg} = 2.9057/0.3389 = 8.6 \text{ minutes}$$

This may, of course, also be read off directly from the graph. The standard deviation is equal to the slope of the line.

This is a typical example of phenomenological treatment of data. A model has not been approached, but the trace has not been produced by mechanical and casual curve fitting (e.g., by a fourth-order polynomial). This is the overture to modeling. (Curve fitting is the overture to interpolation or extrapolation as done in Appendix 2.)

10.24 REFERENCE

Snedocor, G. S. and Cochran, W. G., (1982), *Statistical Methods,* Iowa State University Press, Ames, IA, pp. 385–387.

CHAPTER 11

Iteration

11.1 ONE ITERANT

MANY expressions are such that one parameter is not known. Several cases have already been mentioned, including that of kinetic equilibrium. An example of where iteration would be necessary would be the data for a drying curve such as shown in Table 11.1 and Figure 11.1. Here data are *generated* by considering weight, W, versus time, t, and employing the equation:

$$W - 1000 = (W_0 - 1000)e^{-0.22t} \qquad (11.1)$$

A random experimental error is then imposed on each data point.

The drying curve obviously "levels" off, but at which point? It would seem, visually, that this would happen at a y-value of somewhere between 980 and 1020.

The descent is considered logarithmic, so that one may write.

$$\ln [W - W_\infty] = -kt + \ln [W_0 - W_\infty] \qquad (11.2)$$

When the data are plotted in this fashion, using the stated estimates of W_{inf}, the plots in Figure 11.2 result.

It is seen visually (Figure 11.2) that, of the three, the fit using $W_\infty = 1000$ is the best. The correlation coefficients are shown for the three fits in the last line in Table 11.1. The correlation coefficient is also the largest for this figure but usually is not the best monitor for the "goodness of fit" (Figure 11.3). The standard error of the estimate, s_{yx}, is a better measure. This is shown in Figure 11.4.

The minimum in the s_{yx}-curve is at 978, but there is a fair amount of "flutter" due to truncations in the program. What is surprising is that the value is different from the one that is visually correct ($W_\infty = 1000$).

TABLE 11.1. Data Generated by Equation (11.1) with an Error Imposed.

Time	W	ln[W-980]	ln[W-1000]	ln[W-1020]
0	1250	5.598	5.521	5.438
1	1200	5.394	5.298	5.193
2	1160	5.193	5.075	4.942
3	1120	4.942	4.787	4.605
4	1108	4.852	4.682	4.477
5	1090	4.700	4.500	4.248
6	1062	4.407	4.127	3.738
7	1053	4.920	3.970	3.497
8	1043	4.143	3.761	3.135
Coefficient of Determination, R^2=		0.992	0.994	0.988

A good way, in a graphics program, to determine where the maximum is, is to draw the derivative curve and find the point where it equals zero. This has been done for the data from Table 11.1 in Figure 11.5.

In this case, we then find that the best iterant value is $W_\infty = 997.5$, more in line with the theoretical data, where the niveau should be at $W_\infty = 1000$.

In general, using R^2 as a monitor gives a sharper graph, as seen in Figure 11.3. The fact remains that the two "measures" of goodness differ.

One reason for this (but not the ultimate reason) is that the least squares fit has been obtained by a transformed variable.

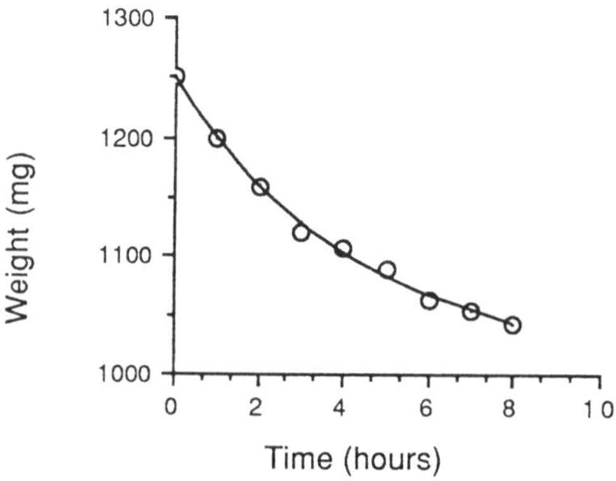

Figure 11.1 Drying curve. Data from Table 11.1.

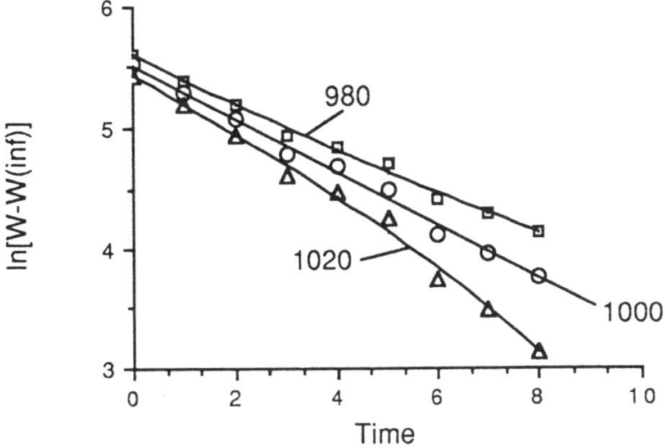

Figure 11.2 Data from Table 11.1 treated by Equation (11.1).

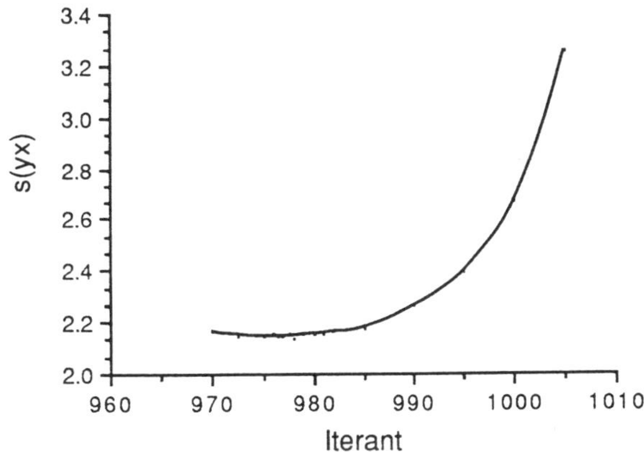

Figure 11.3 Coefficients of determination as a function of iterant.

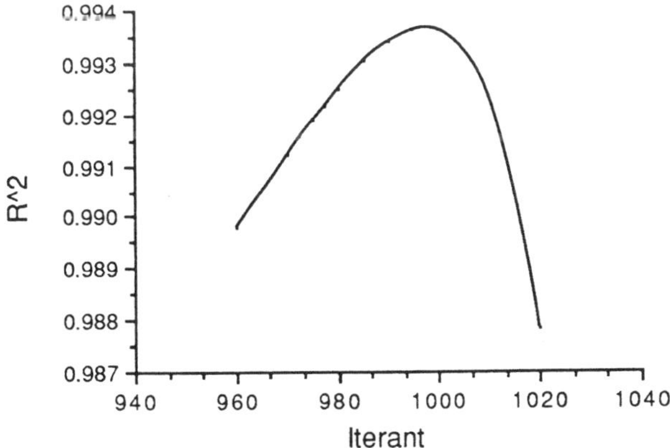

Figure 11.4 Standard error of estimate as a function of iterant.

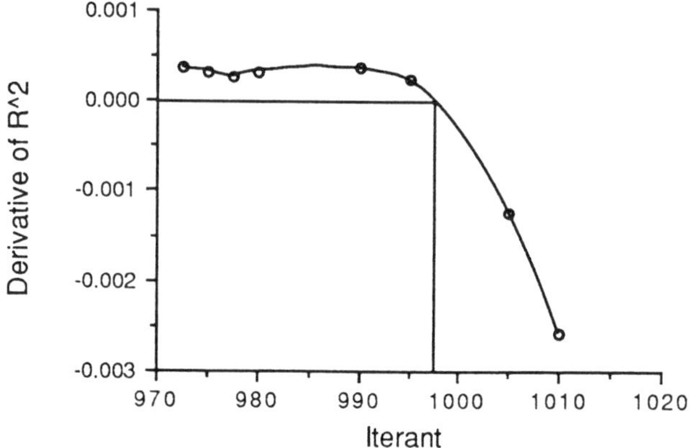

Figure 11.5 Derivative curve of data in Figure 11.4.

11.2 NONLINEAR FITTING

Manually, the correct way of treating such data is to

(1) Obtain a first estimate of the iteration parameter.
(2) Select the criterion for goodness (R^2, s_{yx}, curvature, intercept).
(3) Calculate the criterion parameter value for the first estimate.
(4) Calculate the criterion parameter value for a second estimate, e.g., 10% higher than the first.
(5) Calculate the criterion parameter value for a third estimate, e.g., 10% lower than the first.
(6) Have a statement in the program selecting which "direction" gives the more desirable result.
(7) Repeat (3) to (5) with a parameter value, e.g., 5% lower (or higher as the case may be) or the better iterated value.
(8) Select a criterion for how close two iterated values would have to be before the program should stop.
(9) Print out this value and the pertinent parameters (slope, intercept, correlation coefficient, for instance).

Suppose, for instance, that R^2 were used as a criterion for goodness in the example in Table 11.1. By hand, one would start with, e.g., 1000 as an estimate of a best iterant and then select the higher and lower values as 990 and 1010. One would obtain the R^2-values in Table 11.2.

The program would then deduce that the best value would have to be between 990 and 1010. It would next select 995 and 1005, with the results in Table 11.2 (990, 1000 and 1010 repeated for convenience).

TABLE 11.2. R^2-Values as a Function of Iterant Value.

Iterant	R^2
990	0.99340
995	0.99364
1000	0.99362
1005	0.99325
1010	0.99237

The process is continued (now comparing 995, 997.5, 1000, 1002.5 and 1005). The problem then is when the program should stop. This would have to be done, for example, by asking the program to compare successive values and seek out the two lowest values and ask if they were more than, say, 0.005% different. In the case of 995 and 1000, they are not, and the highest (995) is selected as the best value.

It will be noted that the "precision" of the number obtained is not that good, even if the selection criterion appears to be rather rigid (0.005%). The number could be 999; i.e., there could be a 0.4% error. Also, in the above example, the slopes and intercepts for the two iterant values, 995 and 1000, are shown in Table 11.3.

Most often (as would be the case here), the slope would be the value of interest, and even if there are "precision criteria" of 0.005% in the iteration stop, the iterants themselves differ by about 5% and the slopes differ by 10%.

It is true that nonlinear iteration is more exacting, but there should always be a certain amount of questioning of the "precision" of the values obtained by iteration. Furthermore, the procedure is not very "robust." Slight changes in the experimental data would change the iterant and the slopes considerably.

With prebought programs, some of the problems are

(1) In iteration, it is not necessarily known what parameter is used for the goodness of fit. (In SigmaPlot® this is spelled out.)

(2) It is not a known priori if the program transforms or does not transform the data. (An example is discussed under Polynomials in Chapter 10.)

TABLE 11.3. Iterant Value Effect on Slope and Intercept.

Iterant Value	Slope	Intercept
995	-0.2091	5.527
1000	-0.2201	5.516

Another, even more serious, problem with iteration is that of secondary minima.

11.3 CURVATURE

It has been shown earlier that one way of handling curvature is by means of a polynomial expression, the simplest being a second-order polynomial. The principles of iteration should be applicable to curved data, e.g., data that follow a second-order polynomial. It was mentioned in Chapter 10 that many programs transform variables and obtain parameter values by multiple regression. An example of nonlinear curve fitting via SigmaPlot® is shown below.

SigmaPlot® uses the Marquardt-Levenberg algorithm. It creates the sum of squares of the equation values minus the experimental values and then employs a least squares procedure in seeking a minimum of the sum of squares.

As an example, a set of dissolution data, as they change with storage time, is listed in Table 11.4. The variable is Q_{30}, which is the percent of drug that has dissolved after 30 minutes of exposure to dissolution testing. The first set shows a "precise" set of data, and the second set shows a more realistic set of data.

The program shown in Table 11.5 is placed in a Transform File in SigmaPlot®, and the results in Table 11.4 are entered into the worksheet of the program. It would seem obvious from the data that they level off about 50%, so that an equation of the type

$$Q_{30} = (100 - m)e^{-bx} \tag{11.3}$$

would be applicable. As a first estimate for m, the value 50 is used, and for b, it is noted that the "half-life" would be when Q_{30} is equal to 75, so it is about 3 months. Since now, $k \times 3 = 0.693$, a first estimate of $b = 0.2$

TABLE 11.4. Dissolution Q_{30} Data as a Function of Storage Time.

Storage Time (Months)	Q30 Set 1	Q30 Set 2
0	100	100
3	75	74
6	62.5	60
9	56.25	55
12	53.12	53

TABLE 11.5. Transform for Fitting the Data in Table 11.5.

```
[Parameters]

b=0.2
m=50
[Variables]

x=col(1)
y=col(2)
[Equations]

f=(100-m)*exp(-b*x)
fit f to y
[Constraints]

b>0
m>0
[Options]
Iterations=10
```

would be appropriate. When the program is executed, the results in Table 11.6 are obtained.

It is noted that the estimates are "what one would expect" but that the precision (the high CV-values) is poor in both cases. An increase in number of iterations and step size does not improve the assessment, and it may simply be that the curve format [Equation (11.3)], although intuitively correct, is improper.

11.4 MULTIPLE PARAMETER CURVE FITTING

It has been seen in the previous section that many data sets are amenable to multiple regression. At times, the parameters and their relationships are not quite as apparent, for instance, when data are treated at different levels of the different variables. An example would be that of tableting a product at various machine speeds and measuring the hardness of the tablet as a function of applied pressure at each speed.

Such data could be as shown in Table 11.7. It is obvious that the higher the speed, the softer is the tablet, and the higher the compression pressure, the harder is the tablet. It might be tempting and, in many cases, profitable to simply multiply regress the data, and in such a case, the best fit is

TABLE 11.6. Results from Executing the Data in Table 11.4 with the Program in Table 11.4 (SigmaPlot®).

Ba.	Parameter	Value	Standard Error	CV (%)	Dependence
1	b	5.794e-02	9.803e-03	1.606e+01	0.511
1	m	4.841e+00	4.981e+00	1.029e+02	0.511
2	b	5.973e-02	1.102e-02	1.045e+01	0.506
2	m	5.379e+00	5.811e+00	1.000e+02	0.506

afforded by

$$H = 4.36875 + 0.995P - 0.03105\ [\mathrm{RPM}] \qquad (11.4)$$

P is applied tableting force and RPM is rotations per minute of the die table. To check how such data fit, one may, of course, calculate H manually by inserting all the P- and RPM-values. This task is carried out more easily with a program, as shown in BASIC in Table 11.8. The output is shown in Table 11.9, with the data from Table 11.8 in parentheses for comparison. The fit is fair, at best, and it is actually unreasonable to expect that a linear relationship between H and both P and RPM would exist.

When there is more than one independent variable, it is best to plot the data holding one of the variables constant and repeat this for the other values of the variable that was kept constant. One then gets "best" curves (and getting the "best" parameter values from these curves) for evaluation,

TABLE 11.7. Hardness Profile as a Function of Machine Speed.

Speed (RPM) —> / Applied Pressure (ton)	Hardness (kP) 50	100	150	200
2.5	4.2	3.1	2.5	2.1
5	7.7	5.8	4.6	3.8
7.5	11	8.4	6.7	5.6
10	14.7	11	8.8	7.3

TABLE 11.8. Program for Equation (11.4).

```
100 READ R,P
110 N = N+1
120 Y = 4.36875 + 0.995*P - 0.03105*R
130 PRINT R,P,Y
140 IF N = 16 GOTO 1000
150 DATA 50,2.5,100,2.5,150,2.5,200,2.5,50,5,100,5,150,5,200
160 DATA 5,50,7.5,100,7.5,150,7.5,200,7.5,50,210,100
170 DATA 10,150,10,200,10
1000 END
```

as shown in Figure 11.6. The equations of the lines are obtained from the program, and the slopes and intercepts are shown in Table 11.10.

a and *b* are plotted as a function of speed in Figure 11.7. Note that it is advantageous to present both on one graph. Often, it is necessary to multiply one of the parameters by a factor to make the numbers of the same order of magnitude, but in this case they, by nature, are of the same magnitude.

To observe the curvature, the command "Interpolate" is given in the Cricket menu, and it is seen visually that there is curvature in both of the parameters. This, in itself, negates the rationale for simply using multiple regression.

The most logical approach would be to take logarithms of the *y*-values, and this is done in Figure 11.8. It is obvious from Figure 11.8 that the ln [*b*]-values are linear with speed but that the ln [*a*]-values are curved. Again, observing Figure 11.7, it would appear that ln [*a*] approaches 0.3.

TABLE 11.9. Hardness Profile as a Function of Machine Speed.

	Hardness (kP)			
at Speed (RPM)-->	50	100	150	200
Applied Pressure (ton)				
2.5	5.3(4.2)	3.7(3.1)	2.2(2.5)	0.6(2.1)
5	7.8(7.7)	6.2(5.8)	4.6(4.6)	3.1(3.8)
7.5	10.2(11)	8.7(8.4)	7.2(6.7)	5.6(5.6)
10	12.8(14.7)	11.2(11)	9.7(8.8)	8.1(7.3)

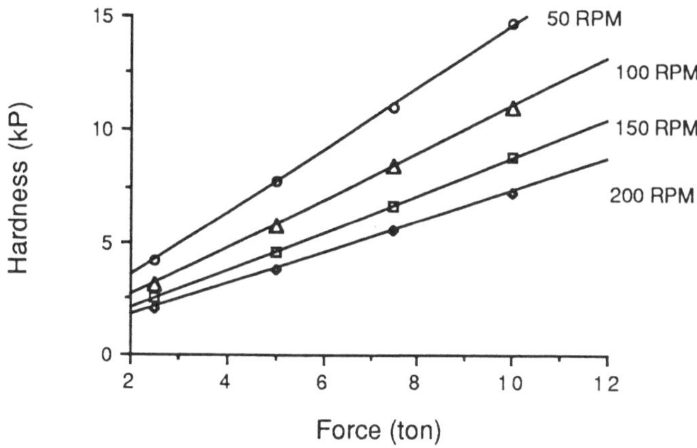

Figure 11.6 Data from Table 11.6.

The plotting is, therefore, carried out logarithmically again but this time using ln $[a - 0.3]$ as shown in Figure 11.9. This is similar to the weight loss problem earlier. It is, of course, best to carry this out by iteration, but for multiparameter plotting, estimates are often sufficient to get an overall good fit. In any event, the estimates will serve as a good first estimate, should it be desired to fit the data nonlinearly.

The best overall fit of the data is

$$H = a + bP \tag{11.5}$$

But

$$a = 0.3 + \exp(-0.223)\exp(-0.03863\,[\text{RPM}]) \tag{11.6}$$

and

$$b = \exp(0.5373)\exp(-0.004609\,[\text{RPM}]) \tag{11.7}$$

so the best overall equation is

$$H = 0.3 + 0.8\exp(-0.03863\,[\text{RPM}]) + \{1.711\exp(-0.004609\,[\text{RPM}])\}P \tag{11.8}$$

TABLE 11.10. Hardness Profile as a Function of Machine Speed.

Speed	50	100	150	200
a	0.7	0.5	0.4	0.35
b	1.392	1.052	0.84	0.696

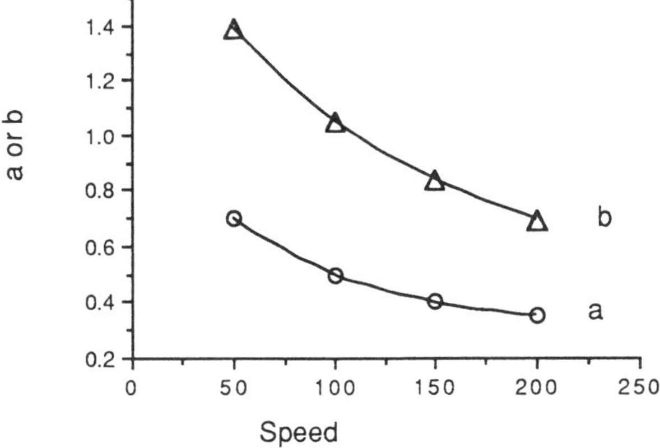

Figure 11.7 Data from Table 11.4.

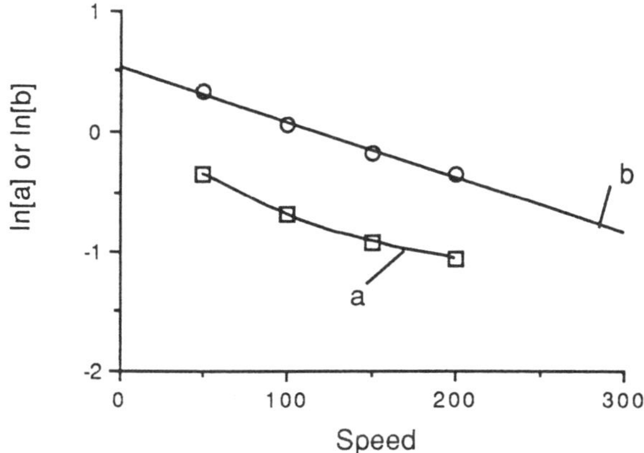

Figure 11.8 Parameters from Figure 11.9 plotted logarithmically. The least squares fit of the b line is $y = 0.5373 - 0.00461x$ ($R^2 = 0.992$)

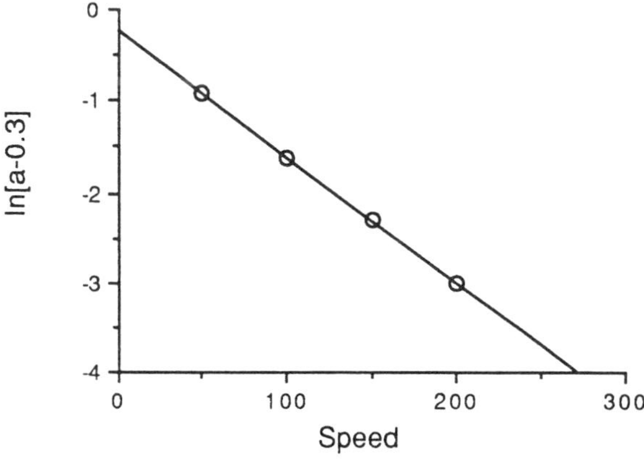

Figure 11.9 The least squares fit is $y = -0.22314 - 0.03863x$.

TABLE 11.11. Program for Fitting Data to Equation (11.8).

```
INPUT "RPM=";A
INPUT "PRESSURE=";P
B1 = 0.3 + (0.8*EXP(-0.03863*A))
B2 = 1.711*(EXP(-0.00461*A))*P
B3 = B1 + B2
PRINT B3.
```

In cases of such fitting, the $y^{\wedge}$-values should always be calculated and compared with the actual data. To do this, it is wisest to write a short program, as shown in Table 11.11 for calculation.

When the experimental RPM- and P-values are inserted in the program, the values in Table 11.12 result. It is seen that the fit is quite good. Further refinement could probably be made by iterating the a-plateau more refinedly.

If it were desired to plot nonlinearly, then one would still have to know the functionality to employ [Equation (11.8)], and so the approach taken above would be a necessary preamble to any nonlinear fitting.

11.5 A PHARMACEUTICAL EXAMPLE (SHEAR CELL)

The data in Table 11.13 are from a powder shear cell. Here, the tangential

TABLE 11.12. Calculated Hardness Profile as a Function of Machine Speed. Experimental Data from Table 11.7 Are in Parentheses.

	Hardness (kP)			
Applied Pressure (ton)	At Speed (RPM)-->50	100	150	200
2.5	3.8(4.2)	3.0(3.1)	2.4(2.5)	2.0(2.1)
5	7.2(7.7)	5.7(5.8)	4.6(4.6)	3.7(3.8)
7.5	10.6(11)	8.4(8.4)	6.7(6.7)	5.4(5.6)
10	14.7(10)	11.1(11)	8.9(8.8)	7.1(7.3)

TABLE 11.13. Shear Cell Data of Powder Compacted to Various Degrees of Densification.

	Tangential Stress			
	Density, ρ (g/cm^3) = 0.8	0.9	1.0	1.1
Normal Stress x 10^{-3}				
1	236	275	316	359
2	308	355	405	457
3	360	413	468	525
4	402	460	518	580
5	438	499	561	626
6	470	534	599	667
7	499	565	633	702

stress needed to move a shallow cylindrical ring containing powder over a similar, stationary ring is tabulated versus the normal stress. The powder can be presented to the apparatus in various densities (by compacting it before the experiment). The task is to find an overall equation that fits the data.

The data are plotted in Cartesian mode on CricketGraph™, and different presentation modes are tried out. Figure 11.10 shows the data fitted by a "logarithmic" fitting mode from the menu.

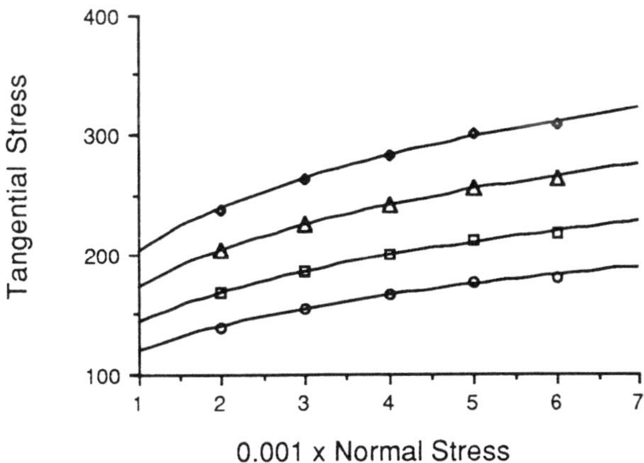

Figure 11.10 Data from Table 11.12.

TABLE 11.14. Parameter Values from Figure 11.10.

ρ	A	n
0.8	236	0.385
0.9	275	0.371
1.0	316	0.357
1.1	359	0.346

It is seen that the data fit nicely to

$$y = Ax^n \tag{11.9}$$

The data are plotted in Cartesian fashion in Figure 11.10, and the values of A and n are shown in Table 11.14 and Figure 11.11.

The least squares fits are

$$n = 0.489 - 0.131D \tag{11.10}$$

$$A = -93 + 410D \tag{11.11}$$

So the overall equation would be

$$y = \exp(410*D - 93)*x^{\exp(0.489-0.131*D)} \tag{11.12}$$

11.6 MULTIPLE ITERANTS

It is, of course, possible to have situations where more than one iterant

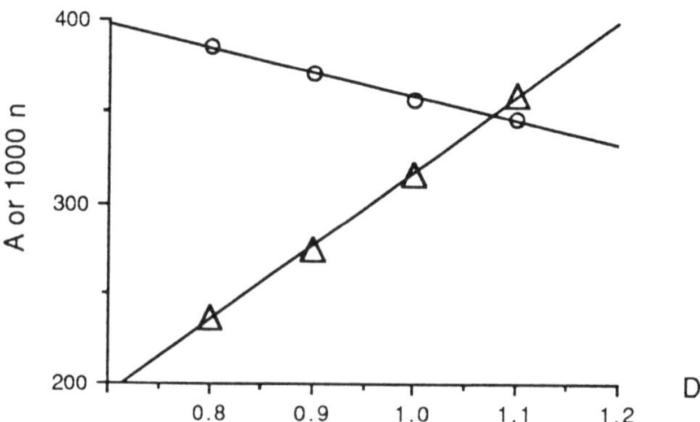

Figure 11.11 A or $1000n$ plotted as a function of density, ϱ.

is at hand. If, for instance, y is a function of x_1 and x_2 and, for the sake of argument, these were associated with constants of unknown magnitude, then we may write

$$y_i = F(x_{i1}, a_1)F(x_{i2}, a_2) \tag{11.13}$$

where we have assumed that the variables are separable (although not necessarily in additive terms). There will be n such equations, and there should exist a value or values of a_1 and a_2 such that

$$\partial\Sigma(y^\wedge - y_i)^2/\partial a_1 = 0 \tag{11.14}$$

and

$$\partial\Sigma(y^\wedge - y_i)^2/\partial a_2 = 0 \tag{11.15}$$

However, there may be several sets of (a_1, a_2) that may satisfy these conditions, and only one will have a smallest sum of squares. One therefore distinguishes between true and false minima.

Powerful programs (such as SigmaPlot®) will, today, allow calculation of the minima, but the "first" estimates must be good. Furthermore, any substantial scatter in the data are likely to cause the program to "cease," i.e., it gives up after a certain number of tries.

The more iterants, the more uncertain are both the type of fit and the parameter values that are obtained. As an example, a blood level curve is generated by the following equation:

$$y = 10e^{-0.5x} + 5e^{-0.1x} - 15e^{-1.4x} \tag{11.16}$$

The data are shown as "Experimental" in Table 11.15.

TABLE 11.15. "Experimental" and "Fitted" Three-Exponential Data.

Time (hours)	"Experimental"	"Fitted"
0	0	0
0.5	7.06	7.094
1	10.34	10.343
1.5	11.74	11.718
2	12.23	12.186
4	11.48	11.468
8	8.95	9.0116
12	6.99	7.0527
18	4.89	4.8828
24	3.47	3.3805

TABLE 11.16. Results of Nonlinear Fitting of the Data in the First Two Columns of Table 11.15.

Parameter	Value	Std.Err.	Dependency
c	-5.00	8.7	0.99
a	1.437	5.0	0.99
d	14.71	0.09	0.90
b	0.0613	0.0007	0.66
q	-9.725	8.7	0.99
m	1.438	2.6	0.99

When the data in the first two columns are subjected to nonlinear curve fitting by SigmaPlot® in the form

$$y = Ae^{-ax} + Be^{-bx} - Ce^{-cx} \tag{11.17}$$

then the results shown in Table 11.16 are obtained.

It might, on the surface, seem that the program has not "done its job" because the parameter values are very far afield from the values from which the data were generated. It should be recalled that the data in columns 1 and 2 are generated; i.e., the errors on this set of data are simply truncation errors.

SigmaPlot® gives the $y^{\wedge}$-values, so both these "fitted" data (shown in the last column of Table 11.14) and the generated ("experimental") values can be compared. Aside from visual inspection, it is instructive to plot the data, and Figure 11.12 shows a plot where the symbols are the generated

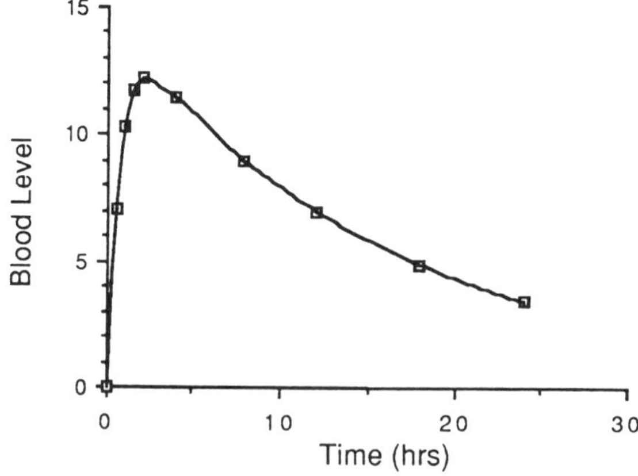

Figure 11.12 Data from Table 11.14. The points are from the second column, i.e., the generated, "experimental" points, and the curve is that generated by nonlinear fitting methods.

"experimental" points and the line constitutes the curve. One could hardly ask for a better fit, yet the parameter values are quite different from the "true" figures.

This illustrates the point that the more parameters, the more "good" solutions are possible. Often, a poor initial estimate will result in the data arriving at a "false minimum." In any event, parameters obtained from iteration of more than two iterants should be viewed with skepticism. So using more than two iterants, although often applied, is a most dangerous practice. It is more worthwhile to attempt to get independent estimates (e.g., during additional experimentation) of some of the iterants.

An example could be a drying experiment with a limiting value of the weight, W_∞, of the powder being dried. Suppose the drying was (and it undoubtedly is) a function of the particle size (diameter d) of the solid.

In this case, the function could be

$$W - W_\infty = (W_0 - W_\infty) \exp[-kt/(d - d^*)] \qquad (11.18)$$

where d^* is a critical diameter, k is a mass and heat transfer coefficient, and t is time. Here, both the "critical" diameter, d^*, and the final weight would be unknown.

11.7 DECONVOLUTION

The term *convolution* (not deconvolution) stems from Laplace transform theory. It often happens that the transform $f(q)$ is known, but the inverse transform $f(t) = \mathscr{L}^{-1}[f(q)]$ is not known. If the transform can be written as a product of two functions with known transform, one may write

$$f(t) = \mathscr{L}^{-1}[f(q)] = \int_0^t \mathbf{g}(s)\mathbf{h}(t - s)ds \qquad (11.19)$$

For instance, if one assumes that the transform for $1/q^3$ is not known, but that of $1/q^2$ ($\mathscr{L}^{-1} = h(t) = t$) and $1/q$ ($\mathscr{L}^{-1} = g(t) = 1$) is, then one may write

$$f(t) = \mathscr{L}^{-1}[q^{-3}] = \int_0^t \mathbf{g}(s)\mathbf{h}(t - s)ds = \int_0^t 1[t - s]ds$$

$$= [ts - (s^2/2)]\Big|_0^t = t^2/2 \qquad (11.20)$$

The result is actually known to be $t^2/2$ in advance from tables of transforms. Note that, in the case of convolution, $f(t)$ is not known, but $\mathbf{g}(s)$ and $\mathbf{h}(t - s)$ are known.

The most common application of deconvolution in the pharmaceutical sciences is to blood level data. In the case of deconvolution, $f(t)$ (the blood level curve after administration of a tablet, for instance) is known, $h(s)$ (the blood level curve after administration of an oral solution) is known, but $g(s)$ (the contribution to the concentration of drug in solution in the stomach) is not known.

Wagner and Nelson (1963) were the first to introduce the concept of deconvolution to pharmaceutics. An example of the utility of this method is shown in Table 11.17, which gives the blood level curves after administration of a solution and after administration of a tablet. It can be shown (see appendix to this chapter) that this may often be simulated by a three-term exponential.

If the solution curve is denoted $h(x)$ and the tablet curve is denoted $f(t)$, then the integral

$$y = f(t) = \int_0^t \mathbf{h}(x - s)\mathbf{g}(x)dx \qquad (11.21)$$

is considered, and now $f(t)$ and $h(x)$ are known, $g(x - s)$ is not. By means of deconvolution, the function $g(x)$, the input function, can be found. This has some importance because, if this input function can be

TABLE 11.17. Blood Level Curves after Administration of a Tablet and a Solution of a Drug Substance.

Time Hours	Solution	Tablet	Time Hours	Solution	Tablet
0	0	0	0.5	5.0	2.75
1	10	5.5	1.5	15.5	9.25
2	21	13	2.5	25.5	18.5
3	30	24	3.5	32.5	26.5
4	35	29	4.5	35.0	29.5
5	35	30	5.5	32.0	28.5
6	29	27	6.5	24.5	24.5
7	20	22	7.5	15.0	19.0
8	10	16	8.5	7.5	13.0
9	5	10	9.5	3.5	7.5
10	2	5			

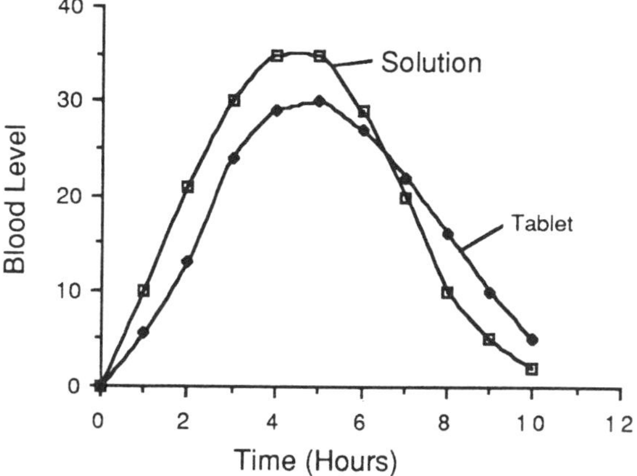

Figure 11.13 Blood level data from Table 11.17.

associated with an exponential with the same exponent as a dissolution curve, then a so-called one-to-one correlation can be established (USP, 1992).

The pharmacokinetic question then is: What is the "dissolution" of the tablet in vivo? As mentioned, the blood level curves after administration of (a) a solution and (b) a tablet are known (Figure 11.13).

The equation for the solution might be

$$h(t) = 40e^{-0.16t} - 40e^{-0.35t} \tag{11.22}$$

If one takes a given point in time, e.g., at $t = 8$ hours, then one may simply calculate the "solution blood level" as

$$h(8) - 8.69 \tag{11.23}$$

If the same impulse, as it is referred to, were administered not at time 0 but at time 5, then the amount released at $t = 8$ would be given by

$$h(8 - 5) = 40e^{-0.16*5} - 40e^{-0.35*5} = 9.20 \tag{11.24}$$

In general, if a fraction of a dose $g(s)$ is released at time s, then the response at time t would be

$$g(s)h(t - s) \tag{11.25}$$

If there were two inputs, $g_1(s)$ at time s_1 and $g_2(s)$ at time s_2, then the response $f(t)$ at time t would be

$$f(t) = g(s_1)W(t - s_1) + g(s_2)W(t - s_2) \tag{11.26}$$

or, in general, if there is a continuum of inputs, $g(s)$, i.e., an input function (the dissolution function), then

$$f(t) = \int_0^t g(s)h(t - s)ds \tag{11.27}$$

Note that the dummy variable is s (not t) and that the integral becomes a function of t (not s) much like Equations (11.20) and (11.21).

If a blood level curve is divided up in intervals, then the integral becomes a summation and may be written as

$$f(t) = \Sigma g(s)W(t - s)\Delta t \tag{11.28}$$

and this type of step function is one way of carrying out deconvolution. Deconvolution is best carried out with special programs.

Sugawara et al. (1994) have reported on successful deconvolution, using a user-friendly, IBM-compatible deconvolution program: NDCREV. In general, the interested reader is referred to the articles by Langenbucher (1982), Chan et al. (1987), and Vaughn and Dennis (1978) for details on "simple" deconvolution. Particularly, the article by Langenbucher is instructive and easy to read.

There are several limitations to the approach (linearity requirements in some of the approaches, equal intervals in others). The programs, however, work fairly well as long as the data are fairly precise, but once there is noise in the data, problems may arise. Podczeck et al. (1995) have used information theory [maximum entropy approach (Shannon, 1948)] to flatten responses and have shown excellent ascertainment of input functions.

11.8 THE LEAST SQUARES WRIST

It is obvious from Sections 11.6 and 11.7 that fitting using many iterants is fraught with danger. An example was mentioned previously where an exponential decay curve, when fit via (logarithmic) transformation, gave rise to erroneous results.

In such cases, it is often advantageous, before trusting the output of the program, to place a pencil in one's hand, bend one's wrist, and draw a smooth curve through the points that seems "reasonable," a least squares wrist.

Points are then taken off this curve and treated by StatWorks™ or SigmaPlot® and the sum of squares extracted and compared to that of the program itself. With the nonlinear fitting program in Section 11.6, it is not the fault of the program, in essence, that the results do not correlate with reality. Indeed, they do correlate with reality, because (in Figure 11.12) the fit is graphically perfect.

11.9 MODELING BY COMPARISON AND STATISTICS

If a researcher does work in a field, and there is ample evidence that the type of quantitative relationship s/he might expect is of a given type, then s/he usually proceeds by plotting accordingly. If one does solution kinetics, the first approach is to plot in log-linear fashion, presuming the reaction to be pseudo-first-order.

It is when deviations occur that researchers attempt better curve fitting and then attempt to explain, e.g., "extra terms," by some molecular or mechanical or chemical attribute. A typical example is adsorption data, which usually fit a BET equation but when higher water activity experiments are conducted, at times, fit the GAB (Guggenheim/Anderson, de Boer) equation.

Sometimes, a series of "models" exist, each associated with a given equation. An example of this is that of Agbada and York (1994), who studied dehydration of theophylline dihydrate and fitted the data to a series (ten) of different equations known to be associated with different models. They then selected the one that fit the best and concluded that the mechanism associated with that equation was the one that applied.

11.10 ZERO-POINT PROBLEMS

A case where $x = 0$ causes problems is the logarithmic transformation of

$$t = Ax^n \tag{11.29}$$

Nonlinear plotting would not suffer from this. If the relation is

$$y = B + Ax^n \tag{11.30}$$

then no such problem need exist (depending on the sign of B and the domain of x).

In the logarithmic plots where zero appears, it is necessary to drop this point. There are many functionalities for which that holds, a notable case being the Gibbs adsorption isotherm:

$$\gamma = A + (\Gamma/RT) \ln [C] \tag{11.31}$$

Here, γ is the surface tension, A is a constant, C is surfactant concentration, T is absolute temperature, and Γ is the surface excess. If made "nonlogarithmic," then nonlinear fitting can often be carried out, but in the case of Equation (11.31)

$$\ln [C] = \Gamma/\{RT[\gamma - A]\} \tag{11.32}$$

now becomes

$$C = \exp(\Gamma/\{RT[\gamma - A]\}) \tag{11.33}$$

This could be nonlinearly fit, but it is seen that it is the inverse function:

$$\gamma = A + [(\Gamma/RT \ln C)] \tag{11.34}$$

which is of interest, and Equation (11.34) still has the zero-point problem. Equation (11.33) might, however, be a better way of obtaining the value of A.

11.11 AN EXAMPLE OF MULTIPLE ITERANTS

The behavior of a gas, e.g., moisture, in the presence of a dry solid is such that a certain amount of moisture is adsorbed, and the amount (volume, v, at standard temperature and pressure, STP) depends on the relative humidity (RH) or the water activity (a = RH/100) of the surrounding atmosphere.

The type of such adsorption isotherms was explained in mathematical terms by Brunauer et al. (1938) based on the following assumption: water is first adsorbed on the solid surface, but before this is completely covered, a second layer starts forming, and before this is complete, a third layer starts forming, and so on. It is assumed that the heat associated with the first layer is H_1, and for all the subsequent layers, it is the heat of condensation of water (H_L = 44 kJ/mole). The equation derived based on this model is the so-called BET equation:

$$a/[v(1 - a)] = [1/(cv_m)] + \{a[(c - 1)/(cv_m)]\} \tag{11.35}$$

where v_m is the volume of water (at STP) covering a monolayer and c is given by

$$c = \exp[-(H_1 - H_L)/RT] \tag{11.36}$$

The assumption made is shown in Figure 11.14. Figure 11.14(a) shows the assumptions in the BET equation schematically.

Since low moisture contents, from a practical point of view, are difficult to obtain when sample sizes are as small as those used in modern, high-sensitivity microcalorimeters, it would be of importance to attempt to establish a correlation between heat and mass transfer. In such a case, it should be possible to directly obtain the traditional isotherm (gram moisture adsorbed per gram of solid versus relative humidity). This can be done by means of a BET equation (Pudipeddi, 1996) but can also be done by an iterative procedure.

It should be noted that there is a paradox associated with this, and that is that, in the limit, there is adsorbed moisture associated with the heat of adsorption of bulk liquid water, yet the pressure about the adsorbent is not equal to the equilibrium pressure ($a = 1$) of water.

This is a natural consequence of the arbitrary assumption in the model that there are *two* heats of adsorption in the process, but it is more rational to assume that it goes down gradually from one high value, H_1 at low coverage, to the "equilibrium" value H_L at high coverage [Figure 11.14(b)]. But this equilibrium, in a true boundary sense, should be the situation where an infinite number of layers have been adsorbed, because only then will the layer truly be like bulk liquid and be associated with a heat of condensation of H_L.

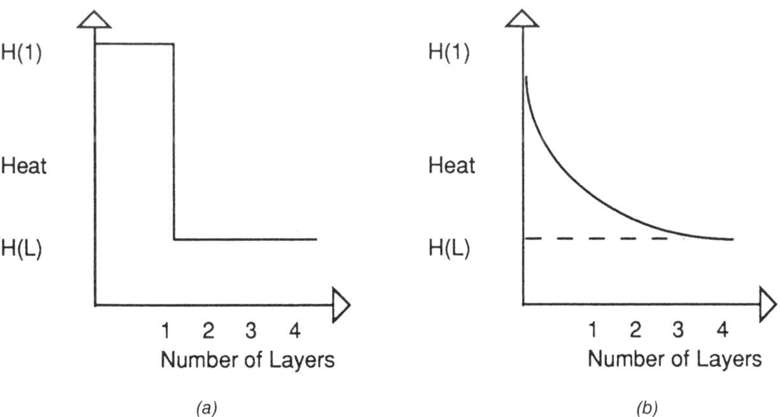

Figure 11.14 (a) Assumption made in the BET model and (b) in the continuous iteration model.

Such a function would be

$$H = H_L + (H_1 - H_L)\exp(-q_1 v) \tag{11.37}$$

where v is the volume (at STP) of water adsorbed per unit mass of solid and q_1 is a constant. The question then is: What is the functional dependence of v on a, the water activity?

It is noted that the above approach is a departure from the BET approach but that the dilemma encountered in the BET approach (solved by assuming two heats of adsorption) has not been resolved, because to tie in Equation (11.35) with a, the water activity, it is necessary to assume a functional relation between the two. This type of approach is denoted an input function approach and will be covered in more detail elsewhere in the text. This differs from the approach used in the BET equation, and (this may seem like a circular argument) the BET equation is assumed to be the best input function.[15]

We may then write an approximate (c being large) BET relationship between v and a by assuming the value of c in Equation (11.35) to be large:

$$(1 - a)^{-1} = q_2 v \tag{11.38}$$

where

$$q_2 = 1/v_m \tag{11.39}$$

The differential form of Equation (11.38) is

$$-(1 - a)^{-2} da = q_2 dv \tag{11.40}$$

Inserting Equation (11.38) into Equation (11.37) gives

$$H_L + (H_1 - H_L)\exp\{-q_3/(1 - a)\} \tag{11.41}$$

where

$$q_3 = q_1/q_2 \tag{11.42}$$

Employing this, we may now write for the total heat, h, adsorbed at a given water activity, a_1:

[15]Input function approaches are common in modeling. Einstein's approach to the heat capacity dependency of temperature is one case; the Prout-Tompkins equation is another.

$$h = \int_0^{a_1} [(H_L + (H_1 - H_L)\exp\{-q_3/(1 - a)\}]dv$$

$$= -\int_0^{a_1} [(H_L + (H_1 - H_L)\exp\{-q_3/(1 - a)\}](1 - a)^{-2}(1/q_2)da$$

$$= H_L(a_1/(1 - a_1)) + (1/q_1)(H_1 - H_L)[e^{(q3/(1-a1))} - e^{q3}] \tag{11.43}$$

This is an equation with three iterants, q_1, q_3, and H_L.

If data are fitted to this equation, then q_2 is found from Equation (11.6), and the isotherm in terms of a can be converted to an isotherm in terms of v.

Isotherm data (via heat or moisture) can now be fitted by iteration to Equation (11.43), and the assumption made in the BET equation can be eliminated. H_L may be assumed to be the heat of liquefaction of water, so that only three iterants (H_1, q_3, and q_1) are needed.

11.12 APPENDIX

An example of tri-exponentials, as demonstrated in Figure 11.12, is the case of blood level curves after oral administration of a solid dosage form. Usually, if a solution is administered, the prevailing differential equations are

$$dG(t)/dt = -k_a G(t) \tag{11.44}$$

and

$$dB(t)/dt = k_a G(t) - k_e B(t) \tag{11.45}$$

where $B(t)$ = amount (not concentration) of drug in blood, $G(t)$ is the amount (not concentration) of drug in the stomach (or GI tract), k_a is the absorption rate constant, k_e is the elimination rate constant, and t is time.

There are assumptions made in this, for instance, that the diffusional equations are based on amounts and not concentrations. This may, on the surface, seem minor, but it should be noted that the concentration may change not only because of absorption, but also because of dilution; i.e., the “volume” of liquid will change with time after administration. Even more severe is the assumption that k_a is a constant. These restrictions do not apply to the term $B(t)$, because the volume of distribution may reasonably be considered constant, but it is emphasized, as well, that the model described is what is known as a one-compartment model.

Nevertheless, the equations have been quite successful in the interpretation of blood level profiles obtained after administration of oral solution-dosage forms. Equation (11.46) has the direct solution:

$$G(t) = G_0 e^{-k_a t} \tag{11.46}$$

Inserting this into Equation (11.45) then gives, after applying Laplace transforms,

$$\mathcal{L}\{dB(t)/dt\} = \mathcal{L}\{k_a G(t)\} - k_e \mathcal{L}\{B(t)\} \tag{11.47}$$

where $\mathcal{L}$ is the Laplace transform of argument s. Noting that $B_0(t) = 0$, the expression

$$\mathcal{L}\{dB(t)/dt\} = s\mathcal{L}\{B(t)\} \tag{11.48}$$

is used on the left-hand side of Equation (11.47). The transform

$$\mathcal{L}\{e^{-ft}\} = 1/(s + f) \tag{11.49}$$

is used on the right-hand side of the equation, so that Equation (11.47) now becomes

$$s\mathcal{L}\{B(t)\} = \{k_a G_0/(1 + k_a)\} + \{k_e \mathcal{L}\{B(t)\}\} \tag{11.50}$$

This rearranges to

$$\mathcal{L}\{B(t)\} = k_a G_0/(1 + k_a)(s + k_e)$$

$$= \{G_0/(k_a - k_e)\}\cdot[(1/(s + k_e)) - (1/(s + k_a))] \tag{11.51}$$

The solution to this is then obtained by taking the inverse transforms:

$$B(t) = \{k_a G_0/(k_a - k_e)\}\cdot[e^{-k_e t} - e^{-k_a t}\} \tag{11.52}$$

This type curve has been studied a great deal in the literature, and many examples of good fits exist.

For the oral solid dosage form, it is obvious that, in the stomach or GI-tract, the amount of mass released is the initial amount of drug, M_0, less the amount, M, retained, so that the rate with which material is released into the stomach, $dG_1(t)/dt$, is the opposite of $dM(t)/dt$, i.e.,

$$dG_1(t) = -dM(t)/dt = k_i A(t) C_s \tag{11.53}$$

In in vitro dissolution, an approximation of the area/time relationship that is often followed is

$$A(t) = A_0 \exp^{-qt} \tag{11.54}$$

where q is a constant. Equation (11.53) now becomes

$$dG_1(t)/dt = k_i C_s A_0 \exp^{-q(t-t_i)} = k_i C_s A_0 e^{qti} e^{-qt} \tag{11.55}$$

The rate with which the drug disappears from the stomach is still given by $k_a G(t)$, so that, overall

$$dG(t)/dt = k_i C_s A_0 \exp^{-qt} - k_a G(t) \tag{11.56}$$

The Laplace transform of this is

$$s\mathscr{L}(G(t)) = Q/(q + s) - k_a \mathscr{L}(G(t)) \tag{11.57}$$

i.e.,

$$\mathscr{L}(G(t)) = Q_1/\{(q + s)\cdot(k_a + s)\} \tag{11.58}$$

where

$$Q_1 - k_i C_s A_{0e^{qt_1}} \tag{11.59}$$

The equation relating to the mass of drug in the blood is still given by Equation (11.45):

$$dB(t)/dt = k_a G(t) - k_e B(t)$$

Furthermore, Equation (11.47) still applies:

$$\mathscr{L}\{dB(t)/dt = \mathscr{L}\{k_a G(t)\} - k_e \mathscr{L}\{B(t)\}$$

If one inserts Equation (11.58) into Equation (11.50), one obtains

$$s\mathscr{L}\{B(t)\} = [\{Q/(s + q)\}(s + k_a)] - k_e \mathscr{L}\{B(t)\} \tag{11.60}$$

or

$$\mathcal{L}\ \{B(t)\} = [\{Q/(s + q)\}(s + k_a)(s + k_e)] \quad (11.61)$$

It is assumed in the following that $q > k_a > k_e$. Equation (11.61) can be anti-Laplaced to

$$B = Q_1[Q_2e^{-k_et} + (Q_3 - Q_2)e^{-qt} - Q_3e^{-k_at})] \quad (11.62)$$

where

$$Q_2 = 1/\{(k_a - k_e)(q - k_e)\} \quad (11.63)$$

$$Q_3 = 1/\{(k_a - k_e)(q - k_a)\} \quad (11.64)$$

These equations are predicted by the sequence $q > k_a > k_e$. Other sequences would change the order of the terms in Equation (11.62).

11.13 REFERENCES

Agbada, C. O. and York, P., (1994), *Int. J. Pharm.*, 106:33.

Brunauer, S., Emmett, P. H., and Teller, E., (1938), *JACS*, 60:309.

Chan, K. K. H., Langenbucher, F., and Gibaldi, M., (1987), *J. Pharm. Sci.*, 76:446.

Kuo, J., Mitchel, D. and Tuerck, T., (1993), SigmaPlot®, Transforms & Curve Fitting, Jandel Corp. No Address, page 7-1.

Langenbucher, F., (1982), *Pharm. Ind.*, 44:1275.

Norby, J., Rubenstein, S., Tuerck, T., Farmer, C. S., Forood, R., and Bennington, J., (1993), SigmaPlot® program creators.

Podczeck, F., Charter, M. K., Newton, J. M. and Yuen, K.-H., (1995), *Eur J. Pharm. Biopharm.*, 41:254.

Pudipeddi, M., (1996), Ph.D. thesis, University of Wisconsin: Use of microcalorimetry in pharmaceutical applications.

Shannon, C. E., (1948), *Bell Syst. J.*, 27:379.

Sugawara, S., Imai, T. and Otagiri, M., (1994), *Pharm. Res.*, 11:272.

United States Pharmacopoeia, (1993), United States Pharmacopoeial Convention, Rockford, MD, 23:1929.

Vaughan, D. P. and Dennis, M., (1978), *J. Pharm. Sci.*, 67:663.

Wagner, J. G. and Nelson, E., (1963), *J. Pharm. Sci.*, 52:610.

CHAPTER 12

Factorials and Phenomenology

CURVE fitting is the simplest first approach to an understanding of what happens in a given situation. Phenomenology is the next more advanced approach and has its start in curve fitting.

The term *phenomenology,* in general, connotes some type of systematic presentation of empirical facts. It goes beyond curve fitting in the sense that one attempts to

(1) Find the exact form of the variables (e.g., $1/T$ K^{-1} in rate constant versus temperature relationships, rather than simple plotting against t°C).
(2) Look for interactions between terms.
(3) In some way, tie in the results with a physically acceptable view. This latter may be, to some degree, mathematical but phenomenology is not strictly *derived.*

To some extent, there is only a thin line between curve fitting and phenomenology, but the fact that deductions are made from phenomenology is the most important distinguishing characteristic.

An example would be the dissolution of a polydisperse powder, such as described by Carstensen and Patel (1975). It was found that the cube root plot was biphasic, and it was deduced that the point where the data transitioned was the point at which the first (smallest) particle had completely dissolved.

In other words, it was not only fitting the data to an equation, but also drawing conclusions from the generated curves and their transformations.

Phenomenology is often tied in with

(1) The use of screening and factorials to gain more than skin-deep acquaintance with a system
(2) Use of factorials to investigate interactive terms
(3) Expansion of simple curve fitting into more complex presentation modes

12.1 THE SIMPLE FACTORIAL

Although factorials were discussed previously, a revisit is in order at this point. Often, through factorials, it is possible to arrive at or assume a linear relationship between variables. If this is the case, then the factorial should be tested for interactions.

The case of the factorial in Table 12.1 is an example of how one can transform experimental data into an empirical equation, which would allow extrapolation to values of a desired magnitude. Here the kinetics of a reaction is studied as a function of (a) pH, (b) buffer molarity, M, and (c) temperature, t (°C).

It might be, for instance, that the experiment was carried out at one set of buffer concentrations, but that an intermediate buffer concentration would be more desirable. Without doing the experiment, could one estimate a priori what the rate constant would be under such circumstances? For this purpose, multiple regression might help arrive at an equation of the type

$$k = a + b\,\mathrm{pH} + c\,\mathrm{M} + qt \tag{12.1}$$

The relationship then may be presented, as a first attempt, as

$$k = -306.25 + 40\,\mathrm{pH} + 11\,\mathrm{M} + 0.665t \tag{12.2}$$

Use of ANOVA will show that the model is "correct" only with 88% confidence, and transformations may, of course, be carried out to improve this. One might suspect that the logarithm of the rate constant would be linear in $1/T$, but this is not done here so that these two transformations should probably have been carried out. But the equationing is carried out for computational convenience. The goal is to make an estimate, and one does the best one can. Using the linear approximation is better than saying: "The number would be somewhere between f and g."

Particularly in computer programs where values might be needed at some point in the program, it is convenient to have estimators in equa-

TABLE 12.1. Temperature and Buffer Effects on Rate Constants.

	Temperature			
		25°C		50°C
pH	M=1	M=2	M=1	M=2
7	11	16	19	5
8	29	41	49	90.5

tional form, since they can be easily programmed. However, there is no guarantee that the responses are linear, and, as shall be seen below, testing for cross-products in the independent variables (interaction, in factorial terms) is advocated.

A two-level factorial essentially does not supply substantial information about interactions, and rather than go through ANOVA, it is easier simply to calculate the "lines" associated with k and proceed from there. This will allow a preliminary probe as to whether pH, M, and T have significant effects. If it is assumed that the rate constant is linear in buffer concentration (which is not unreasonable from general knowledge of kinetics), the following *might* be stated for the rate constants at 25°C and pH 7:

$$k - 11 = (16/11)*(\mathrm{M} - 1) \quad (12.3)$$

or

$$k = 1.45\ \mathrm{M} = 9.55 \quad (12.4)$$

and at the higher temperature:

$$k - 19 = (50/19)*(\mathrm{M} - 1) \quad (12.5)$$

or

$$k = b_2\ \mathrm{M} + b_3 = 2.63\ \mathrm{M} + 16.4 \quad (12.6)$$

It is seen that the slope, b, is greatly affected by temperature, t' °C. If one assumed it to be proportional to temperature (probably not a good approximation, but adequate for the immediately present purpose), then

$$b_2 - 2.63 = \{(2.63 - 1.45)/(50 - 25)\}*(t - 50) \quad (12.7)$$

or

$$b_2 = 2.7t - 132 \quad (12.8)$$

Inserting this into Equation (12.6) now gives

$$k = (2.7t - 132)\ \mathrm{M} + 16.4 = 2.7t'\ \mathrm{M} - 132\ \mathrm{M} + 16.4 \quad (12.9)$$

It is noted that there *is* a cross-term in this, and this can be tested for (and is denoted interaction) in the factorial.

The difference between mere curve fitting and phenomenology here is that the scientist

(1) Applies some general knowledge to the system
(2) Uses assumptions
(3) Calculates interactions that might be deemed to be reasonable or workable
(4) Uses variable transforms that would seem to apply to the situation

The latter point is actually violated in the example but could easily be incorporated (by using ln [k] and $1/T$ transforms).

Frequently the number of variables is large, so that a complete factorial design becomes difficult to handle, and various programs (e.g., Statgraphics Plus 7, Manugistics Inc., Rockville, MD) can be used to search for possible two-factor interactions. Li et al. (1996) for instance have used such programs to effect a Placket-Burman design (Haaland, 1988) to study the effects on formulations with seven variables.

12.2 SCREENING FOR VARIABLES

Before a factorial is carried out, it must be known what the variables are. This is a type of screening where the experience of the formulator/scientist is of importance. An experienced formulator would hardly consider the position of the tablet machine in the room as being a factor (although it might be) but would consider the type and level of disintegrant as being important to the performance of a tablet or capsule product.

In the following, it will be assumed that the variables selected include (not consist of *in toto*) the important variables, and a first task would be to select which are important and which are not. Suppose that the following are considered for the factorial:

- disintegrant, x_1
- tableting pressure, x_2
- moisture level, x_3
- relative humidity in room, x_4
- binder level, x_5

It is noted that, to test these completely, two levels of each are required, so that $2^5 = 32$ experiments would be needed. If the responses (hardness, disintegration) are easily obtainable, this is not an excessive number, and one might find, broadly, that only two of the variables, pressure and disintegrant, are significant effects.

Such significance testing is done as described at an earlier point in this text. It should be pointed out that the success of this and further experimentation entirely depend on the *selection of all the proper variables.* If, for instance, the temperature of the tableting area is of significance, the factorial would not reveal this. *Often, unexpected batch failures are due to ignorance of the importance of a particular variable.* There is no safeguard, other than experience, that will help in the full selection of variables.

Good judgment comes from experience. Experience, in turn, comes from poor judgment.

12.3 MULTIPLE SPECIFICATIONS

As an example of the utility of factorials and multiple regression analysis of experimental data, the following is presented. It is known that, in general, tablet dissolution increases with amount of disintegrant, again, grantedly, not linearly, although this will be assumed below. Also, dissolution (Q_{30} figures) suffers (goes down) with increasing pressure during the tableting operation, again, grantedly, not linearly, but this will be assumed in the following.

What then should be the settings on a machine if it is desired that Q_{30} be above 70% and the hardness above 10 kP? To this end, a simple 2^3 factorial (i.e., the two variables at three levels, eight experiments in all) is carried out. To compress tablets from a given granulation at three pressures is almost routine, so the experimental "difficulty" would be that three batches with different disintegrant levels would have to be made. However, the disintegrant is added at the end, so one granulation divided in three, and three admixtures, is the extent of the processing. The dissolution data are somewhat lengthy (an hour each), but the hardness figures can be obtained in less than 5 minutes each. The results are shown in Tables 12.2 and 12.3.

When multiply regressed (StatWorks™), the following equations result:

$$Q_{30} = 80 - 3P + 10D \tag{12.10}$$

and

$$H = 1.167 + P - 1.25D \tag{12.11}$$

It follows from the requirements that

$$70 > 80 - 3P + 10D \tag{12.12}$$

TABLE 12.2. Multiple Regression of Data in Table 12.1 by StatWorks™.

Data File: Table 12.2 — Dependent Variable: k

Variable Name	Coefficient	Std. Err. Estimate	t Statistic	Prob > t
Constant	-306.250000	105.261950	-2.909408	0.027
pH	39.625000	13.477412	2.940104	0.026
M (Molar)	11.125000	13.477412	0.825455	0.441
t°C	0.665000	0.539096	1.233545	0.264

Data File: Table 12.2

Source	Sum of Squares	Deg. of Freedom	Mean Squares	F-Ratio	Prob>F
Model	3940.593750	3	1313.531250	3.615742	0.123
Error	1453.125000	4	363.281250		
Total	5393.718750	7			

Coefficient of Determination (R^2)	0.730589
Adjusted Coefficient (R^2)	0.528531
Coefficient of Correlation (R)	0.854745
Standard Error of Estimate	19.059938
Durbin-Watson Statistic	1.699477

TABLE 12.3. 2^3 Factorial with Disintegrant Level and Applied Pressure as Variables.

Pressure (ton)	Disintegrant, %	Q_{30} %	Hardness, kP
0	1	75	5
10	1	60	10
15	1	45	15
5	2	85	3.5
10	2	70	8.5
15	2	55	13.5
5	3	95	2.5
10	3	80	7.5
15	3	65	12.5

and

$$10 < 1.167 + P - 1.25D \tag{12.13}$$

Substituting equality signs, Equation (12.12) and Equation (12.13) may be solved to give

$$P < 11.63 \text{ ton} \tag{12.14}$$

$$D > 2.64\% \tag{12.15}$$

which are the critical values.

This would be a first estimate, and running of more batches would then fine-tune these estimates. Such experimentation, with more variables, will also pinpoint whether qualifications can be met in the first place. It is difficult for a production department to live with specifications that can only be met a certain fraction of the time.

12.4 DIMENSIONLESS ANALYSIS

Attempts to correlate parameters take on many forms. One frequently used, nonmodelistic, phenomenological approach is that of dimensionless analysis.

In this type analysis, the dimensions of each variable are noted, and attempts are made to correlate each of them with another variable with the same dimension or with products of variables with the same total dimension. The most famous of these is the Reynolds number, developed for fluid flow.

An example of pharmaceutical nature will be mentioned here, viz., flow rate of powders through orifices. The general pattern is shown in Figure 12.1. It is obvious that the equation for this type of system would be

$$(W - W^*) = -k(d - d^*)^n \tag{12.16}$$

where (d^*,W^*) is the maximum point of the curve and where n is usually equal to 2. Danish and Parrott (1971) have shown that it is the reduced diameter (d/D) that is of importance. D here is the diameter of the efflux tube, so we may then write

$$(W - W^*) = -k'[(d - d^*)/D]^n \tag{12.17}$$

where k' is a new constant different from k. It is known, as well, that, for

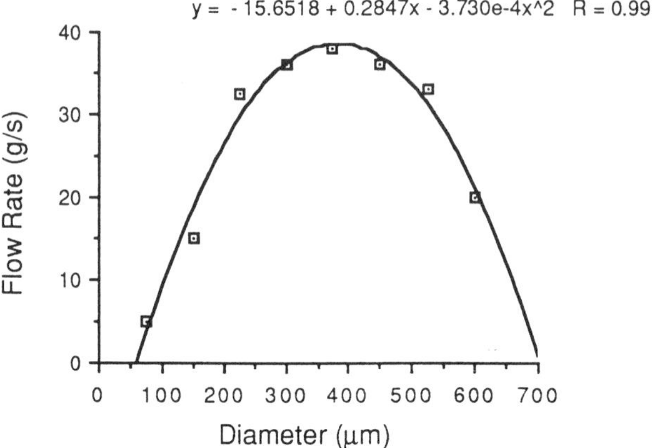

Figure 12.1 Typical flow versus particle diameter plot.

plug flow, the flow rate is linearly related to the length, h, of the efflux tube, i.e.,

$$(W - W^*) = -k''[(d - d^*)/D]^n[a + bh] \tag{12.18}$$

or

$$(W - W^*)/[a + bh] = -k''[(d - d^*)/D]^n \tag{12.19}$$

where a and b are constants and k'' is a constant different from k'.

The flow rate is (or can be) measured in cm^3/sec, so that the dimension of the left-hand side is cm^2/sec—the same dimension as a diffusion coefficient, ϕ. A diffusion coefficient may be obtained from blending studies.

Blending is studied by measuring the standard deviation, s, of a blend after various times. It can be shown (Carstensen and Patel, 1977) to follow the equation:

$$\ln [(s - s_0)/(s - s_\infty)] = -\beta t \tag{12.20}$$

where subscripts denote initial and infinite time conditions. In barrel rolling, β is a function of the internal area of the barrel,[16] i.e.,

$$\beta = \phi/A \tag{12.21}$$

[16]This is not substantiated, except for a few unreported cases. The remaining equations are all drawn from the literature.

where

$$\text{Dim}(\phi) = \text{Dim}(\beta A) = \phi = \text{cm}^2/\text{sec} \quad (12.22)$$

Ω is defined by

$$\Omega = (W - W^*)/\{\phi[a + bh]\} = -k^*[(d - d^*)/D]^n \quad (12.23)$$

and is dimensionless.

$$\ln [\Omega] = \ln [k^*] + n \ln [d/D] \quad (12.24)$$

The quantity that is not known in this equation is ϕ but by means of blending experiments, it may become possible to put the variables in dimensionless form.

Assume that flow and blending experiments were carried out for twenty different materials tested in twenty different hoppers (efflux diameters and efflux tube lengths). One could then calculate the data according to Equation (12.24) and plot the left-hand side for each of the materials versus the ln $[d/D]$ for each of the materials and hoppers. This would give a plot in reduced parameters. Such plots are often found in engineering handbooks and will allow calculation of anticipated flow rates or blending rates for a new, untested material.

The presentation above is idealized, and blending experiments are difficult to carry out with precision, but the derivation serves as an example of how dimensionless parameters could be applied to pharmaceutical systems. This has rarely, if ever, been reported in the pharmaceutical literature.

There are, of course, other approaches. Suppose it were postulated[17] that the flow rate, dM/dt, was proportional to the apparent density, $-M/V$, where M is mass and V is volume.

An equation could then be written:

$$dM/dt = -(k/V)M \quad (12.25)$$

The visualization on the surface may seem quite reasonable,[18] the flow rate being greater, the less densely the powder packs in the efflux tube.

But if such a statement were submitted in a paper, a reviewer would undoubtedly say: With what justification is this assumption made? So it

[17]It should be pointed out that this is the spirit of an example only. The author has no data to show that such a relationship exists.

[18]This is an example only, and the relationship is not correct.

would be challenged by fellow scientists. For what reason should the flow rate have such a relationship to density?

But if we consider the statement carefully, it is no different from saying that the rate of chemical decay (decrease in concentration of a drug in solution, for instance) is proportional to the concentration at a particular time, which is a first-order reaction.

Concepts leading to equations like Equation (12.25) frequently come from looking at curves and saying that, e.g., the flow rate if plotted versus density looks semilogarithmic, and then differentiating the logarithmic equation. But (just like in kinetics) it does not tell us anything about the mechanism. This type of approach is part of phenomenology.

In the case of first-order kinetics, the scientific community automatically accepts it as a reasonable notion, but if applied to another property where it has not been applied before, it raises eyebrows.

12.5 THE DIFFERENTIATION APPROACH

Often, an attempt to "model" a system is to derive a differential equation from experimental data and try to explain the equation loosely in terms of physical phenomena. As an example, consider the kinetic data in Table 12.4.

Such data may be curve-fitted by means of CricketGraph™, and this is done in Figure 12.2. The best fit of the data is to a polynomial of degree 2:

$$C = 99.92 - 0.161t - 0.0414t^2 \tag{12.26}$$

The question we might ask ourselves is whether there is some way of explaining these data. One approach that is a catchall first approach is to differentiate the best equation, i.e.,

TABLE 12.4. Sample Set of Kinetic Data.

Time, t	Percent Retained
0	100
5	98.2
10	93.9
15	87.7
20	80.8
25	70.2
30	57.6

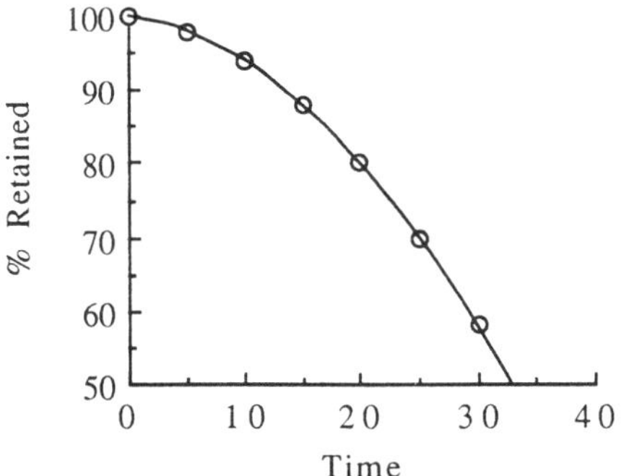

Figure 12.2 Data from Table 12.4.

$$dC/dt = -0.161 - 0.0828t \tag{12.27}$$

To somehow relate this to a kinetic phenomenon, one could postulate that the reaction is zero-order and that the rate constant is time dependent, i.e.,

$$dC/dt = -k$$

$$k = 0.161 + 0.0828t \tag{12.28}$$

But why should the rate constant be time dependent? For that matter, why should the reaction be zero-order? In this type of approach, one, at the onset, does not concern oneself with the real whys in a physical sense, but one simply attempts to find relationships that allow for mathematical explanation of the curves generated.

A publication where this had been done could have as its start of its Results and Discussion section the following wording: "If one assumes that this type of reaction is zero-order, and if one assumes that the rate constant is linear in time. . . ." It does not explain anything, really, and a scientist should not stop at this point. Many researchers do.

This approach also comes under the heading of *input functions* as well, and these will be covered later.

12.6 EXAMPLES OF DIFFERENTIAL FITTING

Assume that the rate of cooling in a given piece of equipment was tested and the data in Table 12.5 were generated.

To use the differential approach, one may enter this in CricketGraph™, ask for a transformation to the first derivative, and obtain the curve shown in Figure 12.3.

TABLE 12.5. Time/Temperature Data for a Piece of Equipment.

Time	Temperature
0	40
10	35
20	32.5
30	31.3
40	30.7
50	30.4

In the program, the data may be fitted in many ways, and the differential curve seems to fit a logarithmic relationship best.

If we assume the logarithmic relationship to be correct (and the treatment is *not* correct[19] here but is presented as an example of how to proceed if no other information or clues are available), we may write

$$-dT/dt = 32x^{-1.7094} \tag{12.29}$$

which integrates to

$$T = [32/(-0.1728)]x^{-0.1728} + I = 45.109x^{-0.1728} + I \tag{12.30}$$

where I is an integration constant. Noting that for $x = 10$, $T = 35$, it

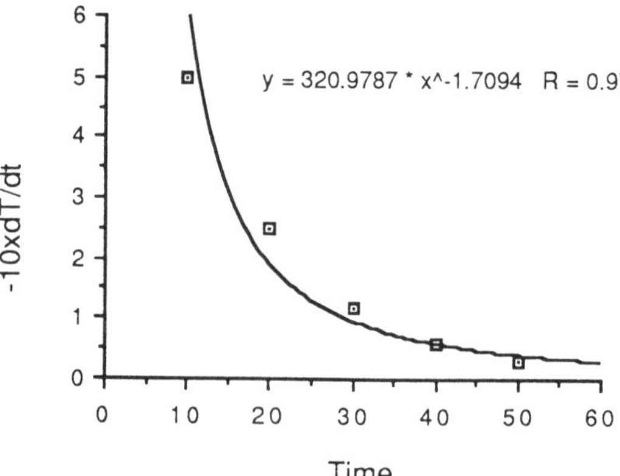

Figure 12.3 Data from Table 12.5.

[19]The reader may recognize this as a set of data that equilibrates at 30°C, i.e., the treatment that follows is basically unsound.

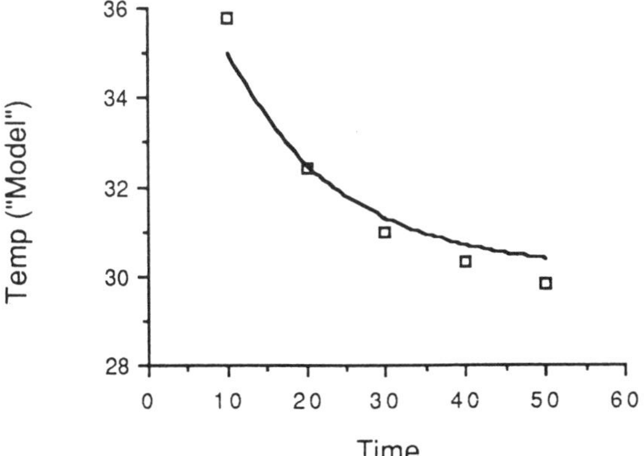

Figure 12.4 Data from Table 12.5. The fitted curve is from Table 12.7.

follows that

$$I = 35 - 45.1 \times 10^{-0.1728} = 27 \tag{12.31}$$

so that the full equation is

$$T = 27 + 45.109x^{-0.1728} \tag{12.32}$$

Generated data using this equation are shown in Figure 12.4 (the curve) with the experimental data from Table 12.5 shown as points.

It is seen that the fit is not too bad. It is obviously not the correct fit, because the temperature has to level off (e.g., at 30°C), but this is presented as an example of what can be achieved and presented in a believable fashion. The graph, of course, can be improved by claiming that the general formula

$$T = A + Bt^{q} \tag{12.33}$$

is what is important and then finding iterated values that fit this equation.

A paper with such an approach would deal with this in the Discussion section as follows: "If it is assumed that the rate with which the temperature, T, decreases is governed by a power-function decrease in time, t, then

$$dT/dt = -b_1 t^{-q} \tag{12.34}$$

This may be integrated to

$$T = b_2 + \{(b_1/1 - q)\}t^{1-q} = b_2 + b_3 t^{1-q} \tag{12.35}$$

where b_2 and b_3 are constants." To achieve some credibility, there should be some explanation as to why the rate should be power-function in time.

It is noted that quite plausible explanations and models may be developed, which are, indeed, simply manipulations of differentiation and integration.

12.7 MONOPHASIC VERSUS BIPHASIC PROFILES

It was shown earlier that, at times, curve fitting of data will result in an apparent curve fit but that, indeed, the curve is biphasic. When such considerations start, then the data treatment falls more in the area of modeling and will be treated later.

A fair amount of almost unethical considerations have been put forth in this chapter. The intent here is, indeed, to show that much phenomenology provides a smokescreen that lets the less astute reader believe that fundamental thinking is involved in the presentation.

There is nothing wrong with phenomenology. It should always be placed up front when assumptions are made, primarily motivated by the production of good fits to data and, in essence, providing explanations that are greatly dependent on the reasonability of the assumptions made.

12.8 OPTIMIZATION

A word on optimization is in order in a text such as this. In short, optimization is arriving at the "best" set of operating conditions for a system. To this, one might add: "with the smallest amount of experiments necessary." It follows from this that abbreviated optimization is rarely exercised in the research mode of investigations. Here, precision and accuracy are not subject to time constraints, at least not if it is serious, investigational research, but in commercial situations, where the "product" is the goal and where containment of cost is of utmost importance, optimization has its place.

The example is a system that is a function of two variables, x and y. The property investigated is denoted z, and the three could be, for instance, related to a tablet that had been difficult to make in the sense that tablets were fairly soft. It should be noted that *at the onset of optimization, a system has already been arrived at,* and the goal is to improve it. In other words, we know at which x- and y-value to start our optimization. Let us assume that the hardness is denoted z, that x is the percent of binder in the formulation, and that y is the percent of disintegrant used. Let us also, for

TABLE 12.6. Response Surface to Equation (12.35).

y—>	3	4	5	6	7	8
x						
3	3.2	5.7(1)	7.2	7.7	7.2	5.7
4	3.8(1)	**6.3**	7.8(1)	8.3	7.8	6.3
5	4.0	6.5(1)	8.0(2)	8.5(3)	8.0(4)	6.5
6	3.8	6.3(2)	7.8	8.3	7.8	6.3
7	3.2	5.7	7.2	7.7	7.2	5.7
9	2.2	4.7	6.2	6.7	6.2	4.7

the point of the exercise, assume that the *true* relationship between x, y, and z is given by

$$z = 8.5 - 0.2(x - 5)^2 - 0.5(y - 6)^2 \qquad (12.36)$$

We shall assume that the formula the formulator has arrived at, the first time he has come up with tablets of reasonable hardness, is such that $x = 4$ and $y = 4$. The critical hardness of the formula, the absolute minimum for performance, is 6 kP, and the formula arrived at has one of 6.3 kP which is rather too close to 6.0 for comfort.

The formulator is unaware of the relationship in Equation (12.35). This equation, if plotted three-dimensionally, is a rounded cone with a maximum at $(x,y) = (5,6)$, and it would be important for the formulator to know this. Rather than drawing a three-dimensional picture, the data in Table 12.6 are generated from Equation (12.35). They show the z-values at different combinations of x and y.

It has to be recalled that our formulator only knows that for $(x,y) = 4.4$,

TABLE 12.7. Response Surface to Equation (12.35).

y—>	3	4	5	6	7	8
x						
2	2.2	4.7	6.2	6.7	6.2	4.7
3	3.2(1)	5.7	7.2(1)	7.7	7.2(3)	5.7
4	3.8	**6.3**	7.8	8.3(2)	7.8	6.3
5	4.0(1)	6.5	8.0(1)	8.5(4)	8.0(4)	6.5
6	3.8	6.3	7.8	8.3(2)	7.8	6.3
7	3.2	5.7	7.2	7.7	7.2(3)	5.7
9	2.2	4.7	6.2	6.7	6.2	4.7

the hardness is 6.3. S/he now proceeds one unit in each direction from this point, the spaces denoted by (1). S/he notices that the value increases when s/he goes up in x and up in y, so s/he goes one unit in each of these directions, denoted by (2), and carries out the experiments. The x-value goes down, but the y-value goes up, so s/he now goes one up in y. The formulator notices an increase (3). A further increase in y makes it go down, and s/he has now improved the performance by 8.5/6.5, or 30%, in eight experiments. More to the point, there is little distance between 8.5 and 6. The basis for this (in a much simplified manner) is the so-called Box method (or EVOP).

Often, a triangular approach is used, and in this case, the sequence would be as shown in Table 12.7. In this case, it took ten experiments, but in many cases, it is advantageous to go by "triangles." The Simplex method uses such an approach.

12.9 REFERENCES

Carstensen, J. T. and Patel, M., (1975), *J. Pharm. Sci.*, 64:1770.

Carstensen, J. T. and Patel, M., (1977), *Powder Technology,* 17:273.

Danish, F. Q. and Parrott, E. L., (1971), *J. Pharm. Sci.*, 60:550.

Haaland, P. D., (1988), *Experimental Design in Biotechnology,* Marcel Dekker, Inc., New York, p. 5.

Li, J. Z., Rekhi, G. S., Augsburger, L. L. and Shangraw, R. F., (1996), *Pharm. Dev. Tech.*, 1: in press.

Natrella, M. G., (1966), *Experimental Statistics,* National Bureau of Standards, *Science Handbook No. 91,* NBS, Washington, DC.

CHAPTER 13

Monte Carlo Method and Simulation

IN real modeling, one visualizes the physical or molecular problem and attempts to describe it in abstract language (i.e., set up an equation), or, failing to do so, one simulates the process by computer (or by hand).

13.1 DESCRIPTION OF THE STEPS OF THE PROCESS

Real modeling usually starts after the scientist has performed a series of experiments and has got some "feel" for the situation. Or it may start with the realization that models proposed in literature cannot be correct or need correction, and hence, once again, some visualization of the process is necessary.

In the worst case scenario, one would not be able to describe the process in abstract language (equations) at all, and that is one of the situations where either the Monte Carlo method or computer simulation is effective.

It is important to state that the first and most important point in modeling is

- to define the physical problem
- to simplify it so it can be handled

13.2 THE INITIAL THOUGHT-PROCESS

Let us assume that we have studied the manner in which pure solids decompose and have found that the decomposition profiles are S-shaped curves. First, the decay is slow; then it accelerates, and then it decelerates.

We might, at first, attempt simply to curve fit these S-shaped curves, and we could come up with several good approaches to the curve fitting:

(1) A cumulative normal (or log-normal) distribution curve

(2) A "titration curve" in the fashion of the Henderson Hasselbach equation

It would probably be possible to get fairly good fits to both, which might afford explanations for the S-shaped curve. With the cumulative distribution curve, if it were normal, it could be that each molecule has an equal chance of decomposing and that it is the average decomposition time (the point at 50% in the curve) that governs the curve and that the standard deviation is simply the standard deviation of this number. (This viewpoint, in fact, is not that different from the one that shall be discussed.) There are two problems with this: first, if it were the case, then the inflection point should always occur at 50% decomposed (which is not always the case), and second, often, the curves do not fit that well to normal distribution curves, but rather to either log-normal or Weibull-type curves.

A rather vague argumentation [a bit like Wagner's (1969) treatment of dissolution curves] could be put forward, assuming the surface exposed is to be log-normal in time; however, it does not help us understand what really goes on.

Here, we would have to visualize various "models." There is no cookbook recipe for how to do that, and often, this step takes time. But let us assume that we started writing down various "models," regardless of how unlikely they might seem. Some means of estimating whether they would lead to reasonable profiles would have to be provided, and often, the model defies mathematical description at the onset.

Some Russian scientists (Gluzman and Arlozorov, 1958), at one time, postulated that a solid always contains a certain fraction of "liquid." Higuchi and Rheinstein (1959) and Guillory and Higuchi (1962), for instance, postulated that this followed a Clausius-Clayperon equation and that the logarithm of the fraction that was "liquid" was inversely related to inverse absolute temperature.

However farfetched[20] that might sound, it is worth developing a model, "just to see." This has not been done here; rather, another (more realistic, but not really that different) view has been adopted.

The model is that the reaction starts at the surface, that there are active sites and decomposition occurs at active sites, and that once a molecule is decomposed, it activates its neighbor(s).

How do we test it if we cannot describe it mathematically? [It has been described mathematically in the literature by Prout and Tompkins (1944), but it shall be assumed here that the process is not known.]

[20] In fact, Ahlneck and Zografi (1990) have suggested "amorphous" regions in surfaces, and whether one calls such regions "amorphous" or "liquid," the concept is the same; i.e., if it were farfetched in 1962, it should also be farfetched in 1995.

13.3 MONTE CARLO METHOD

That the decomposition starts at active sites at the surface, and then works inwards, that is the idea, the visualization. How that is done, no one can tell, although there will be some thoughts put forward in Chapter 16 to this end.

The Monte Carlo method is a good tool for materializing the visualization. One starts out with a grid, like the grid shown in Figure 13.1, which is a 10 × 10 grid (usually larger grids are used), and we shall assign a couple of sites on the periphery (surface) as active sites.

Each square is associated with a two-digit number, e.g., the fifth square in the top row would be denoted "05," and the square in the fourth row and seventh column would be denoted "47." A random number (by table or by computer) approach is then employed to pinpoint places of reaction. A table of random numbers is found in Appendix 9.

To accomplish the reaction, several occurrences may be assumed. It could be assumed that, for instance, the first molecules to decompose were the active sites and that, once they had decomposed, then their neighbors would become active and so on and so on. This makes sense, because it will take a bit of time before the active sites decompose, but in decomposing, they "multiply" so that the acceleratory period is explained. Of course, it has to end sometime, so there will be a deceleratory period as well.

How can we simplify this in such a fashion that it can be handled, can be drawn? Drawing it is exactly what is done (Figure 13.1). The bare grid is simply a 10 × 10 matrix with the rows and columns numbered. A random number table is then employed (or a random number table is generated by use of BASIC and the following program):

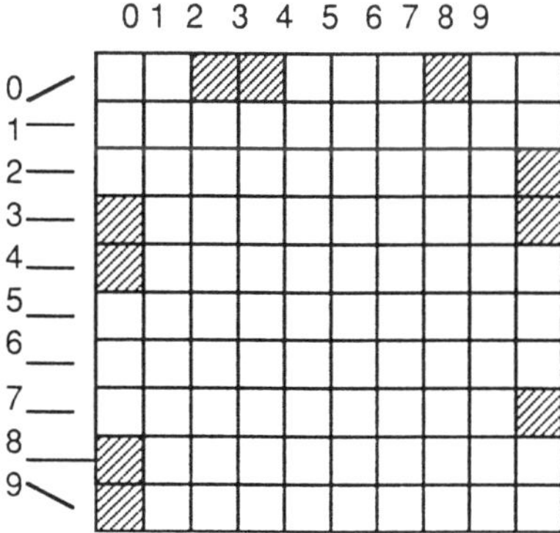

Figure 13.1 Initial Monte Carlo grid showing active sites.

```
INPUT "NUMBER OF 16 DIGIT NUMBERS=";N
FOR Q = 1 TO N
PRINT (10*RND(1)) + 1
NEXT Q
```

Lines 20 to 30 of this program are produced in Table 13.1.

When the RUN command is executed, the screen will display 100 rows of sixteen digits each. (There will be a decimal point that will be disregarded.) We now select a point in the table to start, in this case, row 20. This and the ten next rows read as shown in Table 13.1.

To create a grid with active sites, we first decide, for our first run, how many active sites we want. Ten have been chosen here for convenience (so that the reaction would be relatively "fast"). The first task, then, is to select where the active sites are. For a site to be active, it must be on the "surface," i.e., either begin with zero or nine or end in zero or nine. The first ten numbers encountered in this manner are italicized and underlined in Table 13.1. Once the initial grid has been made up, the "reaction can begin." Hence, time starts at where the break in the table is indicated (at the number 01). In Figure 13.1, these positions are indicated by close cross-hatching.

The rule in the way we visualize this is that, for a molecule to react, it must first be activated, and for it to be activated, it must be neighboring a reacted molecule. We then proceed in the random number table, and the first time we encounter a number that equals that of a "surface site" is the number "79" (boldface). This molecule has now reacted. We note that this has occurred at time 14 and indicate it in the grid in Figure 13.1 by blacking out the square.

We then proceed, and the number "69," a position next to the reacted

TABLE 13.1. Randon Numbers and Monte Carlo Progression.

80	25	72	22	65	24	35	*30*
84	*07*	75	16	*79*	42	*04*	71
76	68	76	79	*29*	07	71	48
55	*39*	40	57	03	54	46	17
43	41	43	29	*09*	82	*97*	12
25	68	53	*02*				
				01	91	19	26
83	62	70	19	02	95	28	93
64	28	**79**	52	18	46	77	12
52	59	*69*	53	46	31	04	25
15	54	48	11	48	17	**97**	88

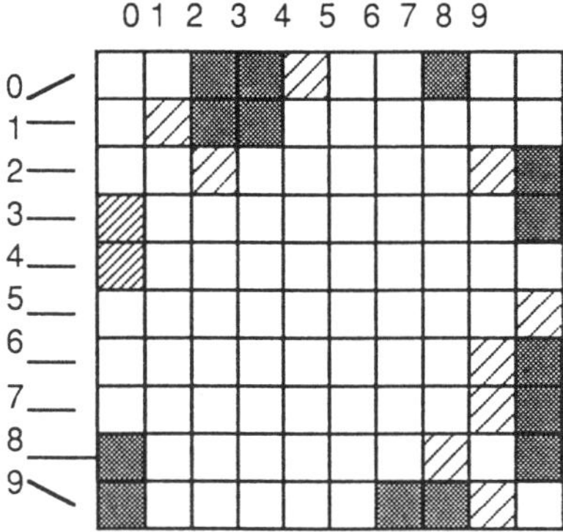

Figure 13.2 Monte Carlo grid after 167 time units.

molecule "79" is encountered after twenty-two time units and is underlined; i.e., it is activated. We make a note of this in our table and our grid.

After thirty-four time units, we encounter the number "97," which was an activated surface molecule, and this is now reacted, and we indicate this in our table and on our grid. We proceed in this manner, and the type of grids in Figures 13.2 through 13.7 result.

We continue the process until the reaction is 85% completed, and a plot is then made of percent decomposed as a function of time (numbers traversed). A curve such as shown in Figure 13.8 results.

It will be noted that, in this scheme, an equation was never written, yet a theoretical trace of the decomposition was arrived at. This can now be repeated with different numbers of active sites, and the effect of the number of active sites on the decomposition patterns is established.

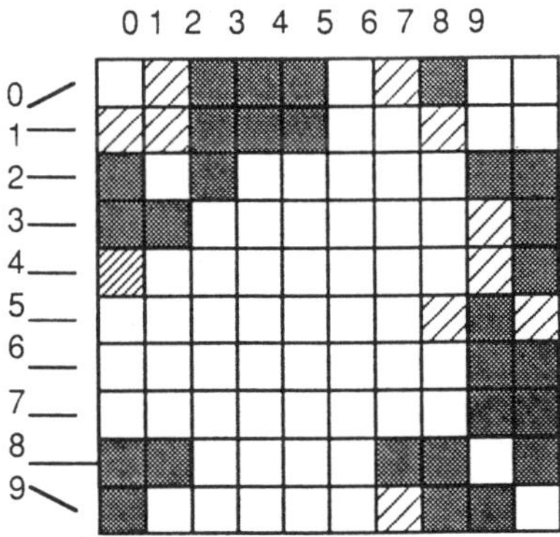

Figure 13.3 Monte Carlo grid after 246 time units.

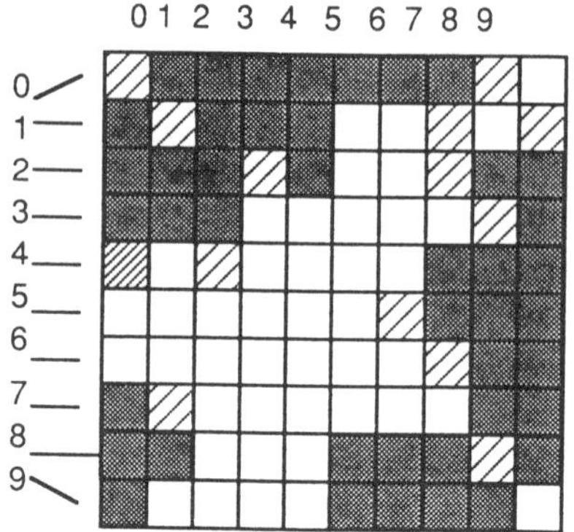

Figure 13.4 Monte Carlo grid after 319 time units.

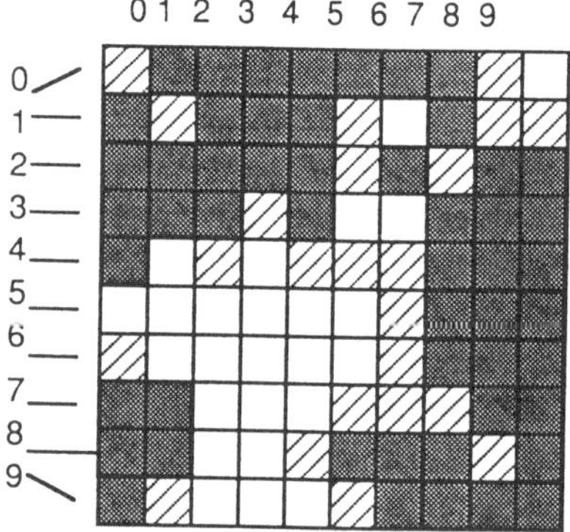

Figure 13.5 Monte Carlo grid after 409 time units.

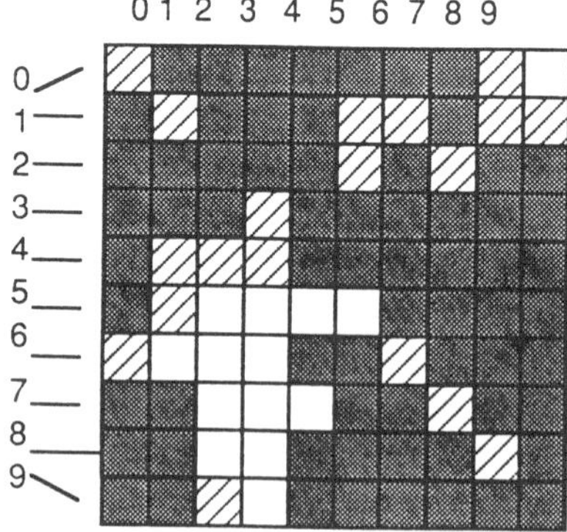

Figure 13.6 Monte Carlo grid after 543 time units.

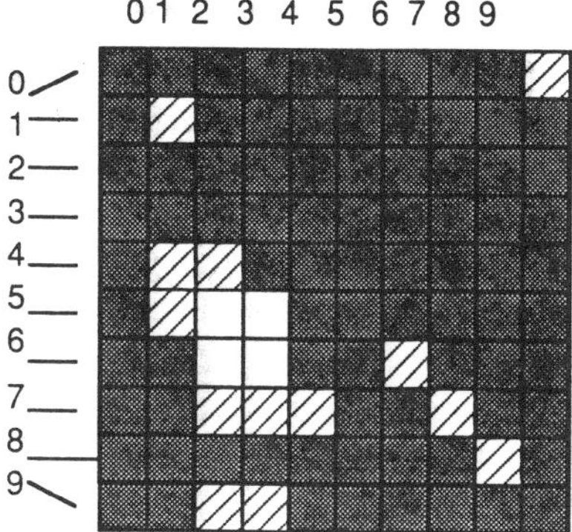

Figure 13.7 Monte Carlo grid after 755 time units.

If the trace is compared with an actual decomposition curve, it would be necessary to multiply the number of times, *N*, by a scaling factor to get the time in the actual scheme, and this ratio then is a measure of the rate constant.

13.4 SIMULATION

Another method that does not apply mathematical principles is simulation. For this, it is necessary to

(1) Visualize the process.

(2) Make assumptions as to how the process progresses.

(3) Write a computer program describing how the first step occurs, leading the program back to where it started, but with the situation as it is

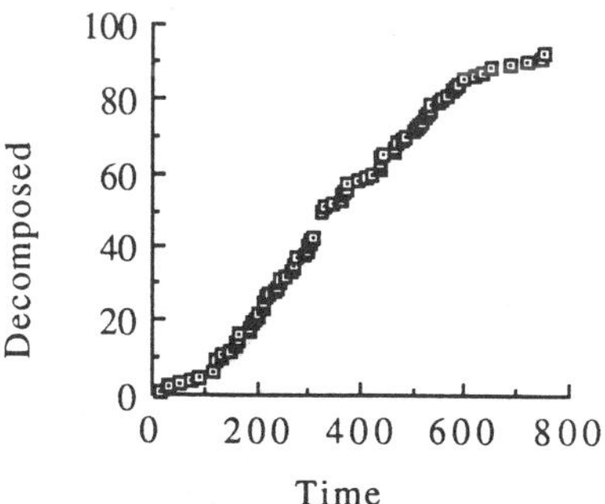

Figure 13.8 Result of solid-state decomposition generated by Monte Carlo method.

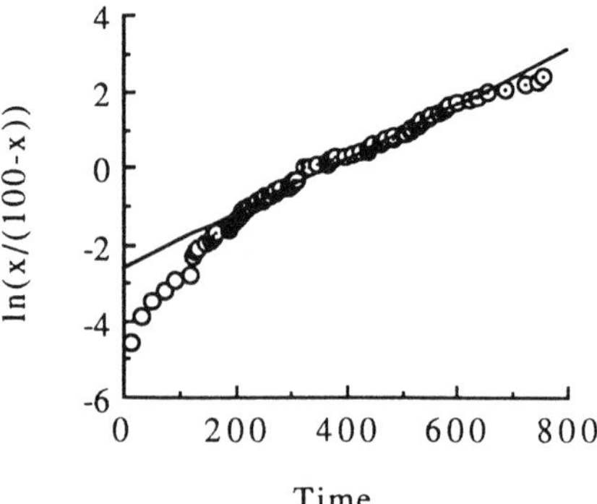

Figure 13.9 Data from Figure 13.8 treated by the Prout-Tompkins equation.

after one step (e.g., one time unit), and to continue the program to a desired point.

Let us assume that we would attempt to describe the dissolution of a particle. One first has to decide how large the particle is, i.e., there must be an INPUT step denoting, for example, the diameter of the particle. This is akin to an *initial condition.*

One next must decide how the particle dissolves. If one says that it dissolves as a function of the surface area, i.e.,

$$\text{Amount dissolved} = \text{constant} \times \text{area} \times \text{time} \tag{13.1}$$

One would have to decide on a time interval; i.e., one starts at time zero, and goes to time Δt and assumes that the area is constant during this interval. One then

- calculates the amount dissolved at time Δt
- recalculates the area after this time unit
- goes back to the initial step

So one has to input a time interval. This is most conveniently done by inputting

- longest time, $T1$
- number of steps, N

and following that with a command stating that the time interval is

$$T2 = T1/N$$

The amount dissolved in a time element, Δt, is proportional to the area, and under sink conditions, to the solubility, S, i.e.,

$$M = qA\Delta tS$$

where q is a proportionality constant. It is convenient to combine the constant and the time to a composite time, t^*, so that Equation (13.2) becomes

$$M = At^*$$

The program, hence, would have the appearance shown in Table 13.2.

It should be pointed out that the Max Time must be small enough so that steps 240 and 250 do not become negative. The program is now run with, for instance, the following inputs:

TABLE 13.2. Program for Simulation of Particle Dissolution.

```
100  INPUT "Density="; D1
110  INPUT "Diameter="; D2
120  INPUT "No of Steps="; N
130  INPUT "Maximum Time=";T1
140  T2 = T1/N
150  PRINT: "Time", "Amt. Remaining"
200  FOR X = 0 TO T1 STEP T2
210  S = S+1
215  REM This is a counter, to stop program eventually
220  Q1 = D1*3.1416*(D2^3)/6
225  REM This is the mass remaining at time X
230  M1 = 3.1416*(D2^2)*T2
235  REM This is the amount dissolved in time T2
240  M2 = Q1 - M1
245  REM    This is the amount remaining after time X+T2
250  D3 = ((6*M2)/(3.1416*D1))
260  D4 = D3^(0.33333)
265  REM This is the new diameter
270  D2 = D4
275  REM   This brings the nomenclature back to Step 230
280  IF S = N GOTO 1000
285  REM   This ends the program
290  GOTO 300
300  PRINT X, Q1
310  NEXT X
1000 END
```

TABLE 13.3. Output from Table 13.2 with the Given Initial Conditions.

"Time"	Amount Remaining	ln[Amt. Remaining]
0	0.524	-0.647
0.01	0.492	-0.709
0.02	0.462	-0.772
0.03	0.433	-0.837
0.04	0.406	-0.903
0.05	0.379	-0.970
0.06	0.354	-1.039
0.07	0.330	-1.110
0.08	0.307	-1.183
0.09	0.284	-1.257
0.1	0.264	-1.333

- density = 1
- diameter = 1
- no. of steps = 10
- max time = 0.1

and the output in Table 13.3 results. The first two columns of the table are shown graphically in Figure 13.10.

It would be natural to curve fit these data logarithmically, as done in Figure 13.11, and it is seen that the fit is quite good. However, true modeling of the situation would show that the correct curve function is that the cube root of the amount remaining is linear in time.

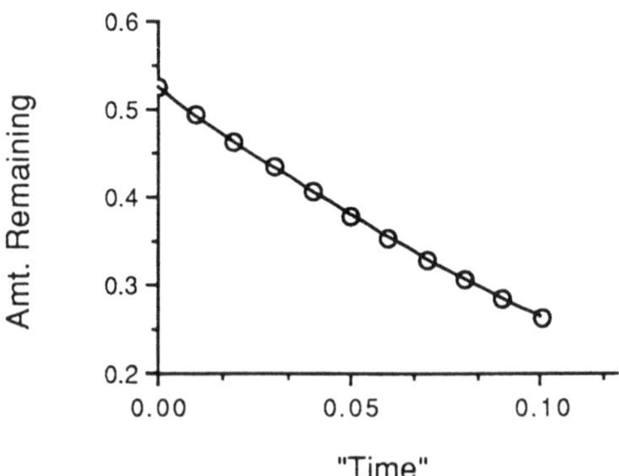

Figure 13.10 Data from the first two columns of Table 13.3.

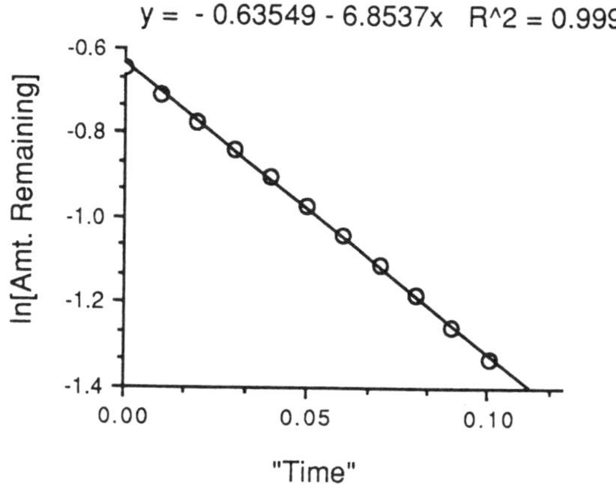

Figure 13.11 Data in Figure 13.10 treated semilogarithmically.

13.5 REFERENCES

Ahlneck, G. and Zografi, G., (1990), *Int. J. Pharmaceutics,* 62:87.

Gluzman, M. and Arlozorov, D., (1958), *Zh. Prik. Khim.,* 31:657.

Guillory, K. and Higuchi, T., (1962), *J. Pharm. Sci.,* 51:100.

Higuchi, T. and Rheinstein, T., (1959), *J. Am. Pharm. Assoc. Sci. Ed.,* 48:136.

Prout, E. and Tompkins, F., (1944), *Trans. Faraday Soc.,* 40:448.

Wagner, J., (1969), *J. Pharm. Sci.,* 58:1253.

CHAPTER 14

Pseudomodeling

PSEUDOMODELING entails some degree of modeling in the sense that previously published models might apply to the situation at hand. It, furthermore, entails situations where existing models do not quite apply to the data at hand and that corrective terms are then added to equations.

14.1 RELYING ON PREVIOUS MODELS

An example of this is recent work on dehydration kinetics. Excellent articles by Agbada and York (1994) and Pudipeddi et al. (1995) are examples of this. In the work by Agbada and York, for instance, a table of existing equations for solid-state phenomena, including the mechanism, is presented. The data are then fitted to each of these equations, and by means of statistical evaluation, the equation that fits the best is assumed to present the mechanism at hand.

The data in Table 14.1 presents a set of data for a polymorphic transformation from a different source. For simplicity, let us assume that this may be presented by either an activated site process (Prout and Tompkins, 1944) or by a stochastic process (Carstensen and VanScoik, 1988). The question then is whether statistical or other treatment of the data will reveal if the process is stochastic or diffusional.

It is seen from Figure 14.1 that the resulting curve is S-shaped. This could result if the process is one of two published models for such processes. As mentioned, either the process could be dictated by activated sites (Prout and Tompkins, 1944) or by the fact that, once nucleation occurs, conversion is (too) rapid (to measure). Hence, the amount converted equals the amount nucleated, and this might be normally distributed about a mean nucleation time. In the former case,

$$\ln [(1 - x)/x] = -k(t - t_{0.5}) \quad (14.1)$$

TABLE 14.1. Kinetic Data for a Polymorphic Transformation.

Time	Fraction (1-x)	ln[x/(1-x)]	Normal Z-value
0	1		
10	0.993	4.95	-2.46
20	0.982	3.99	-2.1
30	0.953	3.01	-1.675
40	0.84	1.66	-0.95
50	0.5	0	0
60	0.269	-1.00	0.615
70	0.119	-2.00	1.18
80	0.047	-3	1.675
90	0.018	-4.01	2.1
100	0.007	-4.96	2.46

where x is fraction decomposed and $t_{0.5}$ is the half time. This treatment is shown in the third column of Table 14.1 and in Figure 14.2.

In the stochastic case, x should be normally distributed; i.e., employing the table in Appendix 1 and calculating the Z-value corresponding to the fraction (column 2 in Table 14.1) and plotting it versus time should result in a straight line. The Z-values are shown in the last column of Table 14.1, and the data presented in this form are shown in Figure 14.3. It is seen, quite clearly (statistical treatment is actually not necessary in this case), that, in this latter case, the data are not linearized; hence, by deduction, it is the former process that applies.

The method distinguishes between known models. It is important in this respect to check for linearity, because this is often much more telling than the sum of the residuals. For instance, the presentation in Figure 14.2 is still not quite linear (deviations being +, −, +), and it may be that a third, yet unthought of, model might apply.

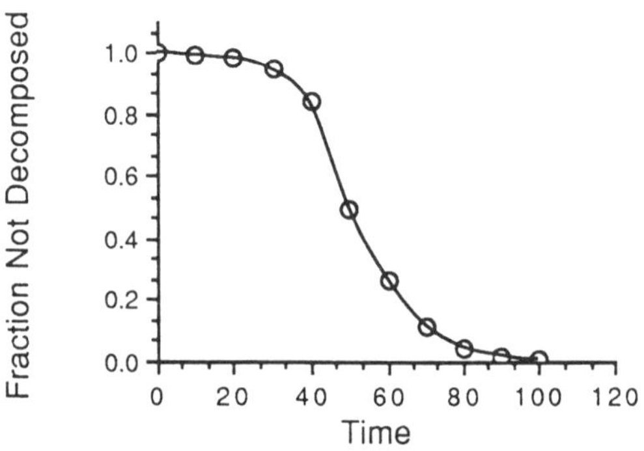

Figure 14.1 Data from Table 14.1 plotted as is.

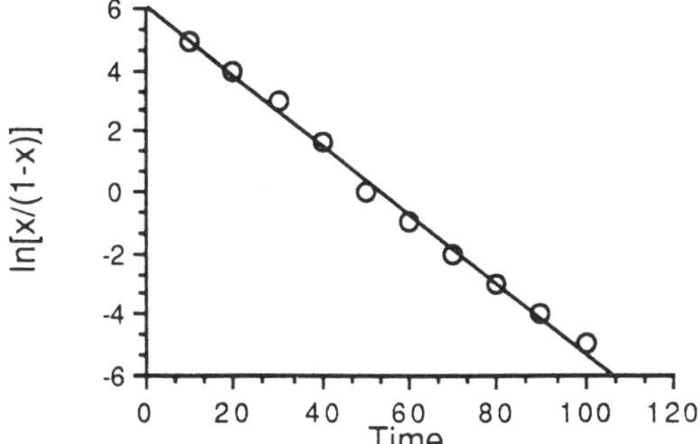

Figure 14.2 Data from Table 14.1 plotted according to activated site method. Least squares fit is $y = 6.107 - 0.113x$ ($R^2 = 0.995$).

14.2 PSEUDOMODELING

We have arrived at the point where we start thinking about modeling, not only conceptually, but also in more mathematical terms, in the sense that we attempt to derive equations from conceptional visualization of the process at hand. In general, it is desired to express "results" of modeling in equation form. In some instances, such "results" are not really the result of attempting to elucidate the system on a "molecular" basis, to use a much overused phrase, but rather to deduce some of the equations that apply "a step back" in the process.

In other cases, a simple first equation is assumed and approximative assumptions are added. Finally, there are cases where *ab initio* equations

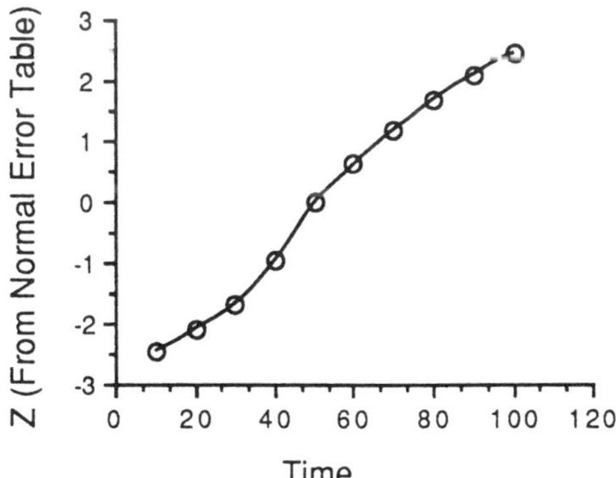

Figure 14.3 Data from Table 14.1 plotted according to the assumption of the process being strictly dictated by nucleation (followed by fast conversion). The nucleation should then be normally distributed around the "average" time.

are arrived at, but these cannot be solved in closed form and are either solved by graphical integration or use of input functions.

14.3 GOING BACKWARDS

It has been seen in the previous chapter that data may often, to great advantage, be fitted to a curve. This allows for interpolation and extrapolation, which, in itself, is quite convenient. The curves obtained in themselves do not say much about what goes on in the physical sense, and in many cases, the curves are simply approximations of the "true" relationship related to the process on a molecular or a microscopic level.

A curve, symbolically, has the equation:

$$y = f(x)$$

where to each x-value, there is one and only one y-value. This may be differentiated, expressed symbolically as

$$y' = f'(x) \tag{14.2}$$

This, at times, relates to the microscopic phenomena, which one may then assume and present one's introduction (not model) in the reverse order; i.e., say that it is reasonable to assume that $y' = f'(x)$ so therefore $y = f\{x\}$. This has been discussed to some extent in Chapter 12.

There are many examples of this in literature. Relating to the log-probability curve fitting of dissolution of tablets, Wagner (1969) worked backwards, and since the dissolution rate is proportional to area, then, if the area generated were a log-frequency function, the integrated curve should be a log-probability function.

This is denoted reverse deduction in this text. It really casts no light on the actual problem but is often useful. As mentioned earlier and repeated here: it may surprise the kinetics reader that every time he states that a reaction is first-order, s/he is actually saying: "I am assuming that the reaction rate, $-dC/dt$, is proportional to the concentration, C, left at time, t":

$$dC/dt = -kC \tag{14.3}$$

and this integrates to

$$\ln [C/C_0] = -kt \tag{14.4}$$

where C_0 is the initial condition. It takes something like a Lindeman hypothesis to show a model to be consistent at a molecular level, with the result in Equation (14.3). The thought process from Equation (14.3) to (14.4) is simply reverse deduction, and it is used so much that it is often confused with true modeling.

Another case, quite akin to the one above, is the Heckel equation (Heckel, 1961), where the investigator had curve-fitted porosity (ϵ) of compacts with applied compression pressure, P, and found that

$$-\ln [\epsilon] = -kP + q \tag{14.5}$$

where k and q are constants. He presented the "model" in reverse fashion by saying that, if one assumes that the rate of porosity change at pressure P is proportional to the remaining porosity, then the differential equation is

$$-d[\epsilon]/dP = -k\epsilon \tag{14.6}$$

It is seen that this thought process is quite analogous to Equation (14.4), which, of course, integrates to Equation (14.6).

14.4 GENERAL EQUATIONS IMITATED IN REVERSE DEDUCTION

The following is a list of the types of reverse differential equations that will lead to curve-fitted equations:

(1) $\ln [M/M_0] = -kt$
- Diffusion: $dC/dt = -DA(dC/dx)$
- Challenge is to find dC/dx
- First-order kinetics: $dC/dt = -kC$
- Convert to fraction, x, decomposed and plot $\ln [1 - x]$ vs. t

(2) Contracting geometries
- $x/x_0 = \{1 - (k/l_0)t\}^n$
- $n = 2$ (contracting cylinder)
- $n = 3$ (contracting sphere)
- Take any linear dimension (a) and state that it decreases linearly in time. These "look" like first-order plots.

(3) Square root plots
- Washburn and Higuchi Equations $a = kt^{1/2}$. These are square root in time. They look like first-order plots. They are variants of contracting geometry.

(4) Probability plots. Weibull plots, log-probability plots
- Diffusion or random phenomena
- The Wagner or Lippmann approach uses the reverse deduction process; example: Wagner (1969), Lippmann (1974).

(5) pH-titration plots, probit plots
- Auto-catalysis; example: solid-state decomposition
- $\ln [x/(1 - x)] = y$

14.5 A PHARMACEUTICAL EXAMPLE: AUTO-OXIDATION

Take the example of an oxidation reaction:

$$R + O_2 \rightarrow R^* \tag{14.7}$$

It is found that the decomposition is a sigmoid curve and, hence, might follow:

$$\ln [x/(1 - x)] = k(t - t_i) \tag{14.8}$$

Plotting shows that this is correct. Now by differentiating Equation (14.8), Equation (14.9) is obtained:

$$dx/dt = k(1 - x)x \tag{14.9}$$

One might now claim that the decomposition is both a function of the amount of drug substance remaining $(1 - x)$ and also (catalytically) by the amount of decomposition product (x) formed. Or the decomposition rate constant is directly proportional to $(1 - x)$.

It is now possible to present the process in reverse order, with the assumption first, leading to Equation (14.9) and from this to deduce Equation (14.8) and then show that the data follow the equation. The author of this book has utilized this approach (Franchini and Carstensen, 1994).

14.6 CURVES WITH EXTREMA

If a profile has a maximum, it is, of course, possible to simply curve-fit it and let it go at that. But some reflection will indicate that, for an extremum to occur, there must be opposing effects, $Q(x)$ and $P(x)$. Their nature may be investigated via the first derivative, which should equal zero at the extremum:

$$dY/dx = 0 = Q(x) - P(x)$$

so that $Q - P = 0$ at the x-value where maximum occurs.

TABLE 14.2. Hardness/Pressure Data (Compression Profile) for a Granulation.

Pressure (kP)	0	2000	4000	6000	8000
Hardness (kP)	0	6	9	10.5	11.25

14.6.1 EXAMPLE 14.1

Assume the data in Table 14.2 relating the hardness of a tablet as a function of applied pressure, and find a pseudomodel for this by reverse deduction.

14.6.2 ANSWER

The data are plotted in Figure 14.4 and fitted to a polynomial equation.

$$y = 235.7 = 3.064x - 0.00022x^2 \tag{14.10}$$

If this is differentiated, then

$$dy/dx = 3.064 - 0.00044x \tag{14.11}$$

One might now "claim" that the rate with which hardness is increased by increased pressure unit applied will decrease from a certain value (b) at the onset and that this rate of decrease is proportional to the pressure (by a factor of $-c$). Hence,

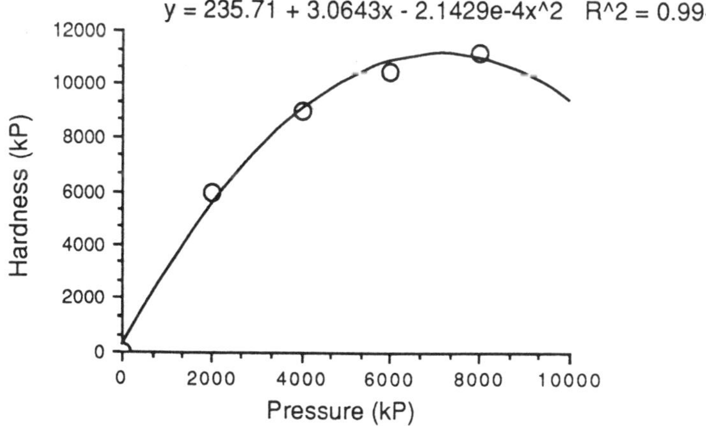

Figure 14.4 Data from Table 14.2 plotted and curve-fitted.

$$dy/dx = b - cx \tag{14.12}$$

where b and c are constants. If this is integrated, then

$$y = a + bx - (c/2)x^2 \tag{14.13}$$

As noted in the graph, this "model" holds, with the values of $a = 235$, $b = 3.06$, and $c = 0.00022$.

All of the curve has been "explained," except for the number 235. In essence, this number should be zero (no hardness at zero applied pressure), but some "suitable" explanation can probably be found. For instance (please note that this author does *not* endorse such interpretations), it may be speculated that the "model" only applies after full consolidation of the powder has occurred, i.e., at a given applied pressure. Or one may show statistically that the intercept is not significantly different from zero.

It is noted that the "conclusions" are arrived at by reverse deduction, and although this works in some cases, in many cases it does not because, most often, the equations arrived at from curve fitting are approximations of actual curves. The best example of this is that, fortuitously, most powders appear to be log-normally distributed. If the process is investigated on the molecular level, then the equations generated produce traces that are approximately log-normal, but it is nonsense to try to derive the equations from the log-normal distribution. In fact, it is not possible.

14.7 MODELS WITH FUNCTIONAL ASSUMPTIONS

Although the use of input functions is most rationally treated under modeling, it may be instructive to introduce the concept with an example at this point.

Often, a model is arrived at mathematically, except that, at one point in the development, a function appears that cannot be expressed in closed form or that cannot be predicted. In such cases, one often resorts to inputting a function simply on the basis that it meets the initial and boundary conditions of the problem.

Sometimes, there is only a vague difference between input functions and assumptions. A famous example is Einstein's heat capacity law where it is assumed that all the molecules vibrate at the same frequency. The model admirably explains the heat capacity of a solid at low and high temperature. (It took thirty years before Debye derived an equation without this input function, or assumption.)

A famous example, which is clearcut as far as input function is concerned, is that of the Prout-Tompkins equation, where the propagation probability, α, is said to be positive at time zero, equal to the termination probability, β, at the inflection of the S-shaped curve and zero at infinite time. There are several such functions, and the simplest one was selected.

There are differences between assumptions and input functions, however, particularly in reverse modeling. If one considers the Wagner approach (Wagner, 1969) to tablet dissolution, one is faced with the assumption that the area generated during dissolution is log-normal in time. There is no precedence for this, and this is clearly an assumption.

Take, on the other side, the Grant equation (Grant et al., 1984), which explains why there may be curvature in a solubility-temperature plot, which usually is linear by the equation:

$$\ln [S] = -(\Delta H/RT) + Q \tag{14.14}$$

where ΔH is heat of solution, S is solubility, R is the gas constant, T is absolute temperature, and Q is a constant. The equation obviously assumes that ΔH is constant; however, there is ample evidence that this is often not true. ΔH is often represented by power series, i.e.,

$$\Delta H = a + bT + cT^2 \tag{14.15}$$

where a, b, and c are constants. Inserting this in Equation (14.14), one obtains

$$\begin{aligned} \ln [S] &= -((a + bT + cT^2)/RT) + Q \\ &= (a/R)(1/T) + \{(b/R) + Q)\} + cT \\ &= (q/T) + q_2 + q_3 T \end{aligned} \tag{14.16}$$

Many pharmaceutical solubility-temperature plots follow this equation, e.g., that of Pudipeddi et al. (1995). The difference between the pure assumption previously cited and this case is that there is ample evidence in other cases that Equation (14.15) holds. The explanation for Equation (14.15) may be considered a different subject for explanation elsewhere.

14.8 MODELS WITH INPUT FUNCTIONS: A PHARMACEUTICAL EXAMPLE

The following example, in a way, leads into the concept of modeling, but fits in well at this point. Suppose, as a very simple example, that one were to model the migration of a drug from the liquid fill of a soft shell capsule

TABLE 14.3. Migration of Drug into a Soft Shell.

Time (hours)	Concentration in Fill
0	80
2.5	54
4	41
5	31
7	24
8	19
9	14
11	10
12	6
14	3
15	0

into the shell. A set of experimental data are shown in Table 14.3 and Figure 14.5.

One would assume that this would be a diffusional phenomenon, and from literature, one would deduce that the amount left in the core liquid, M, and the amount in the shell, $M_0 - M$, would be related by a function of the type:

$$dM/dt = -(DA/h)[C_i - C_s] \tag{14.17}$$

where C_i is the concentration in the fill at time t and C_s is the concentration in the shell. A is the internal surface area of the capsule, and h is the "diffusion film thickness." If two different volumes, V_1 and V_2, are assumed for

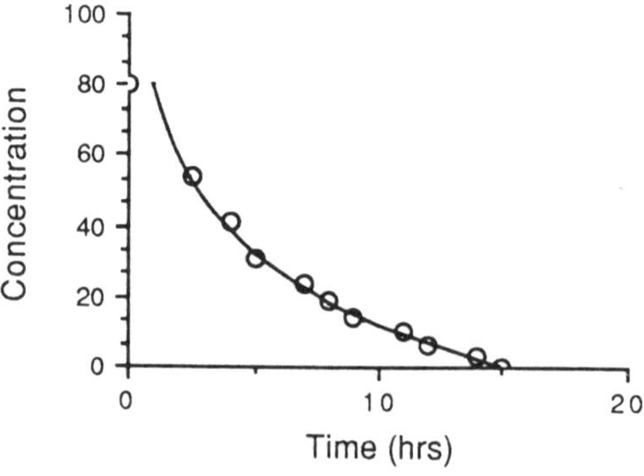

Figure 14.5 Data from Table 14.3 plotted in linear fashion.

fill and shell, then Equation (14.14) can be written

$$dM_i/dt = -(DA/h)[(M_i/V_1) - \{(M_0 - M_i)/V_2\}]$$

$$= -(DA/h)\{(1/V_1) - (1/V_2)\}\{M_i - a\} \quad (14.18)$$

where

$$a\{(1/V_1) - (1/V_2)\}M_0 = M_0/V_2$$

or

$$a = 1/[(V_2/V_1) - 1] \quad (14.19)$$

Since the shell volume, V_1, is smaller than the fill volume, V_2, it follows that a is positive. Equation (14.18), when integrated, becomes a first-order expression and should plot log-linearly in time:

$$\ln [(M_i - a)/(M_0 - a)] = -(DA/h)\{(1/V_1) - (1/V_2)\}t \quad (14.20)$$

The fit is obviously wrong, and if an iterant (a) is imposed on M_i (as shown), then the fit does not improve. Other explanations have to be sought, and it may be argued that h is not constant. For simplicity, if one assumes that the volume of the shell and fill are the same, V, then Equation (14.17) becomes

$$dM/dt = -(DA/Vh)[M_i - (M_0 - M_i)] = -(DA/Vh)M_0 \quad (14.21)$$

Equation (14.21) is absurd in the sense, that, on casual inspection, it predicts that the rate of diffusion is constant. The point is that what is incorrect in the reasoning. The obvious point of attack in such an analysis is the assumptions. There are several assumptions made in Equation (14.17) and (14.21): It is probably correct to assume that A is constant, but is h constant? And is D constant? And what is the effect of the two volumes being the same?

If one assumes that D does not change, then the only remaining term that may not be constant is h. One would now have to state (correctly) that the drug diffuses into the shell and that h is related to the depth of penetration. Since knowledge of h essentially assumes that the equations have already been solved, one is faced with a dilemma.

One then often assigns a function, a so-called input function, which meets the initial and boundary conditions of the problem. In this case, one might state that, at time zero, $h = 0$ and that, after 15 hours, $h = h_c$, the thickness of the capsule. Let us assume this to be 0.2 cm. Hence,

$$h = 0 \text{ at } t = 0 \tag{14.22}$$

$$h = 0.2 \text{ at } t = 15 \tag{14.23}$$

A simple-minded equation that meets these criteria is a linear approximation, i.e.,

$$h = (0.2/15)t = 0.013t \tag{14.24}$$

In this case, Equation (14.22) takes on the form:

$$dM/dt = -(DA/Vh)M_0 = -Q/t \tag{14.25}$$

where

$$Q = DAM_0/(0.013V) \tag{14.26}$$

Equation (14.25) integrates to

$$M = M_0 - Q \ln [t] \tag{14.27}$$

Data from Table 14.3 are presented in this mode in Figures 14.6 and 14.7.

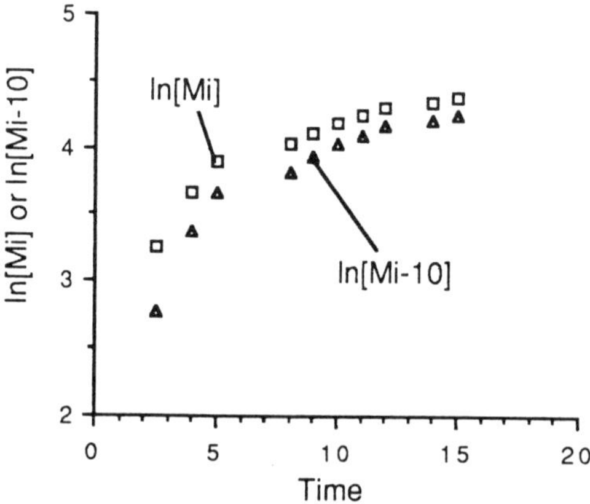

Figure 14.6 Data in Table 14.3 treated semilogarithmically.

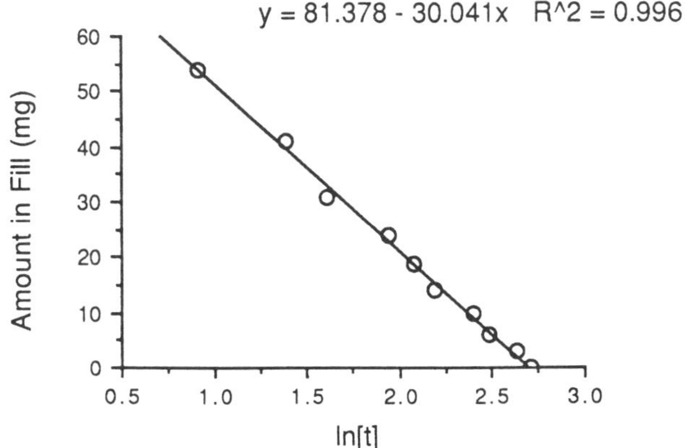

Figure 14.7 Data from Table 14.3 plotted according to Equation (14.17). Least squares fit is: $y = 81.4 - 30x$ ($R^2 = 0.996$).

It is seen that the fit is good ($R^2 = 0.99$) but that there are problems at low time points, since the intercept is 81.4, not 80. Equation (14.17), of course, suffers from, like many equations, (e.g., the Gibbs isotherm) the fact that it is undefined at $t = 0$. Further refinements can then be made by using different values for V_1 and V_2.

One might also refine the model by assuming other input functions that also meet the stated boundary and initial conditions, e.g.,

$$h = h_\infty(1 - e^{-qt}) \tag{14.28}$$

However, with input functions, the simplest possible is the best, since one has no *real* justification for the actual choice.

14.9 ARRIVING AT DIFFERENTIAL OR OTHER EQUATIONS NOT SOLVABLE IN CLOSED FORM

At times, a model is set up and the resulting equation cannot be solved. In that case graphical integration is resorted to. A program in BASIC for integration is shown in Table 14.4.

The function integrated is the Ng equation (Ng, 1972) for the rate of solid decomposition (dx/dt) as a function of remaining intact drug (x):

$$dx/dt = kx(1 - x)^p \tag{14.29}$$

TABLE 14.4. Graphical Integration Program in BASIC.

```
100 INPUT "number of steps=";N1
100 PRINT "Number of steps="
110 INPUT "Rate Constant=";K1
110 PRINT "Rate Constant="
115 INPUT "Maximum Decomposition"; Q1
118 REM When Fractions are used this is 1.0
120 Z = 1/N1
130 PRINT "Time", "Decomposition"
200 FOR X1 = 0 TO Q1 STEP Z
205 M = M+1
210 X2 = (1-X1)^(.3)
220 X3 = K1*X1*X2
230 X4 = X3^(-1)
240 X5 = X4*Z
250 Y = Y + X5
255 Q2 = 10*X1
260 FOR J = 0 TO 10 STEP 1
255 IF Q2 = INT(J*Q1) THEN PRINT Y, X1, J
260 NEXT J
270 GOTO 290
290 NEXT X1
500 END
```

where p, in the program, is set equal to 1/3. To carry out the integration, Equation (14.29) is recast as

$$dx/\{x(1 - x)^{1/3}\} = kdt \tag{14.30}$$

When this program is used with 10, 20, and 30 steps, then Table 14.5 results.

It is obvious that the method gains in refinement with the number of steps, and as known from integral calculus, the integral is defined as the limit of a series with the number of steps approaching infinity.

Above a certain (large) number of steps, the values will be the same, but with the program as written, this would require reams of paper. In order to avoid this, a set of steps is inserted in the program, which allows for the printing of only a fraction of the calculated values. This program is shown in Table 14.6.

Integration programs are available in more sophisticated languages than BASIC, e.g., in SigmaPlot®.

14.9.1 EXAMPLE 14.1

Suppose we were analyzing a dissolution profile of a powder. It is known

TABLE 14.5. Output from Table 14.4 with Different N-Values.

Fraction Decomposed	Time (hours) 10 Steps	Time (hours) 20 Steps	Time (hours) 30 Steps
0	0	0	0
0.1	10.3	15.3	18.6
0.2	15.7	21.5	25.2
0.3	19.4	25.5	29.3
0.4	22.3	28.6	32.4
0.5	24.75	31.2	35.0
0.6	26.95	33.4	37.3
0.7	29	35.5	39.4
0.8	31	37.5	41.4
09	33	39.7	43.6

(Hixson and Crowell, 1931; Carstensen and Musa, 1972; Brooke, 1973; Carstensen and Patel, 1975) that such powders dissolve by way of a cube root dissolution law. Figure 14.8 and Table 14.7 are examples of such behavior, but we shall, for the moment, ignore that we are aware of this.

Let us assume that we dissolve $M_0 = 50$ mg of powder in $V = 900$ ml of water in a USP dissolution apparatus.

14.9.2 ANSWER 14.1

As mentioned, these data follow a cube root equation, but we shall assume that we do not know this, and we shall assume that we set up the dissolution equation:

$$dM/dt = -kAC \tag{14.31}$$

where A is the surface area at time t. C, of course, is the amount dissolved divided by the dissolution volume, V. If the amount not dissolved is M,

TABLE 14.6. Program Allowing Only a Few Values to Be Printed.

```
260 FOR J = 1 TO 10
270 IF T= INT(J*T1/10) THEN PRINT T,x
280 NEXT J
290 GOTO 300
300 NEXT X1
500 END
```

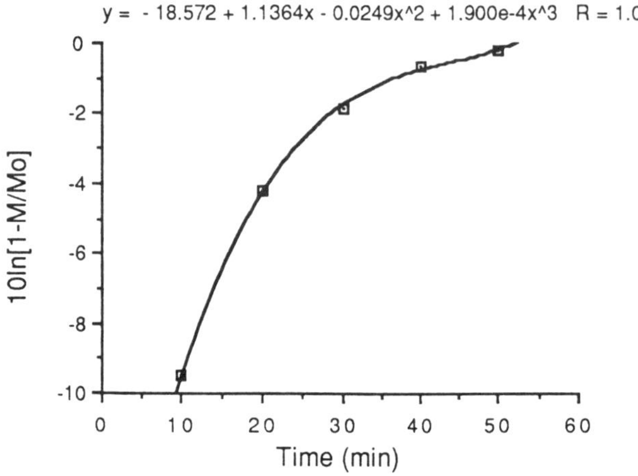

Figure 14.8 Data from Table 14.7.

then

$$C = M_0 - M \tag{14.32}$$

and we can now rewrite Equation (14.30)

$$-d(M_0 - M)/(M_0 - M) = -(k/V)Adt \tag{14.33}$$

The left-hand side is $-d \ln [M_0 - M]$, and on the surface, integration should be simple, except the area, A, is not constant.

In such situations, it is often advantageous to assume a function that will satisfy the boundary conditions. An approach would be to express the area as a power function in time. This is the input function.

TABLE 14.7. Powder Dissolution Data.

Time (min)	mg. Dissolved
0	0
10	19.294
20	32.85
30	41.681
40	46.800
50	49.219
60	49.950
70	49.990

$$A = A_0 + 2at + 3bt^2 \ldots \qquad (14.34)$$

where the coefficients 2, 3, and so on have been included for convenience for the subsequent integration. Equation (14.34) satisfies initial conditions since, at $t = 0$, it is the original surface area, A_0, and it can become zero at some time, depending on the coefficients to the powers to t. Equation (14.33) now becomes

$$-d \ln [M_0 - M] = -(k/V)(A_0 + 2at + 3bt^2 \ldots)dt \qquad (14.35)$$

Higher order terms have been shown by dots. Equation (14.35), when integrated and subjected to initial conditions, becomes

$$\ln [1 - M/M_0)] = (k/V)\{A_0 t + at^2 + bt^3 \ldots\} \qquad (14.36)$$

If $\ln [1 - (M/M_0)]$ is plotted versus t, then Figure 14.8 results, and it is seen that terms of order above two are not necessary in the description of A as a function of time.

It is noted that, in this type of modeling, one arrives at an approximate relationship because one cannot express the differential equation completely correctly, but rather in an approximate fashion.

It is also noted that the derivations have a certain aura of "difficulty" giving the less astute readers the impression of their being sophisticated. But often the simpler a derivation is, the better, and the simpler the model is, the better. The cube root derivation, aside from being more correct than the above, is also much less complicated.

In any event, the example was shown to exemplify the use of an input function in a pharmaceutically oriented case.

14.10 REFERENCES

Agbada, C. O. and York, P., (1994), *Int. J. Pharm.*, 106:33.

Brooke, D. (1973), *J. Pharm. Sci.*, 62:795.

Carstensen, J. T. and Musa, M. N., (1972), *J. Pharm. Sci.*, 63:273, 1112.

Carstensen, J. T. and Patel, M., (1975), *J. Pharm. Sci.*, 64:1770.

Carstensen, J. T. and VanScoik, K., (1988), *Pharm. Res.*, 7:278.

Franchini, M. and Carstensen, J. T., (1994), *Int. J. Pharmaceutics*, 111:153.

Grant, D. J. W., Mehdizadeh, M., Chow, A. H.-L., and Fairbrother, J. E., (1984), *Int. J. Pharmaceutics*, 18:25.

Heckel, R. W., (1961), *Trans. Metal Soc. of AIME*, 221:671.

Hixson, A. W. and Crowell, J. H., (1931), *Ind. Eng. Chem.*, 23:923.

Lippmann, I., (1974), in *Dissolution Technology,* Eds. Leeson, L. and Carstensen, J. T., *The IPT Section of the Acad. Pharm. Sci.*, pp. 193–194.

Ng, W. L., (1972), *Aust. J. Chem.*, 28:1169.

Prout, E. G. and Tompkins, F. C., (1944), *Trans. Faraday Soc.*, 40:489.

Pudipeddi, M., Sokoloski, T., Dudu, S., and Carstensen, J. T., (1995), *J. Pharm. Sci.*, 84:1236.

Wagner, J., (1969), *J. Pharm. Sci.*, 58:1253.

CHAPTER 15

Modeling

TRUE modeling is a step further along than pseudomodeling, in that once finished and presented, it will start with the steps shown below.

15.1 DEFINITION OF MODELING

(1) Visualizing the phenomenon being studied
(2) Expressing this in mathematical terms
(3) Arriving at either an equation or a differential equation describing the data
(4) Showing that the data fit the equation

In addition to this, it may be added that, in modeling, after the first model(s) has (have) been developed, the system is "stressed" to see if reasonable variations in the circumstances (temperature, pressure, for instance) will make the model stand up or falter.

15.2 GETTING STARTED

Usually, modeling starts after some data have been accumulated in a given system, and the scientist asks the question *why?* In some cases, they are an industrial project where, at one point, the scientist again asks him/herself: *why?* In some cases, a literature search or maybe the knowledge base of the scientist will automatically lead her/him in the right direction when s/he is working on a "new" project, but it will be assumed that an entirely new type of data set and experimentation and system are being dealt with and that no direct background information is available.

The presentation to follow is quite informal, and it is purposely kept so.

In modeling, there are ideas, thought processes, failures, successes, and further failures. It is difficult to set up a blueprint for something creative. But what the author has done is to go through a modeling scheme in much the same way it came about twenty years ago.

15.3 LITERATURE SEARCH

Modeling then deals with how to get ideas. Again, a lot of reading is recommended because there is similarity in approaches. Furthermore, a good search is necessary anyway, because references will have to be supplied eventually, and it is also advantageous to find out as soon as possible into the project whether or not the system has been published on before. There is nothing as embarrassing as presenting something as new when it has already been published before. Such events are not all that uncommon. A famous example is that of Heckel (1951) who "reinvented" the Athy equation.

But let us assume that the literature bin was empty, that there were no clues in the literature as to how to proceed. Then one must resort to thinking out the system for oneself. In so doing, one, of course, draws from previous knowledge. Nothing under the sun is completely new.

Different researchers probably have different ways of getting started, but this author usually "doodles" at the onset. A type of drawing of the system is made and discarded in favor of another one, and all along, equations are developed. In other words, a series of models are tried out before an adequate one is arrived at.

The word *adequate* is used because a prerequisite is that the data fit the model. The words *correct* and *true* are not used because *a model is never proven true, simply not proven untrue.* It is always possible that someone later may come up with a better model. When this happens, the second scientist should always give credit to the first one. Science is a progression, where one scientist has ideas that are, in a certain manner, tied in to publications of an earlier day, even though not necessarily directly.

15.4 THE BASIC IDEA

It is best to describe the basic data with an example[21]. Let us say that we are checking the hygroscopicity of a compound by exposing it to various relative humidities. Above a certain relative humidity, strong moisture pickup is recorded, and we might stop right there and say: "This drug

[21]This is based on work reported by Carstensen (1977).

should be kept in areas below 45% RH." The data we may have accumulated may look as shown in Table 15.1.

The experiment is a simple one, and it has a practical purpose: At what ambient conditions can the drug be processed? So far, no modeling is in sight at all. But if the scientist/formulator is asked exactly that question, s/he can do one of two things: (a) run more experiments, (b) try to figure out from the data at what RH pickup starts, or (c) do both, i.e., calculate a critical RH and then substantiate it experimentally.

15.5 GRAPHING

It cannot be emphasized enough that *it is always profitable to graph data.* Even if there seems to be no good reason, even if the prospect is only one of idle preoccupation, it is advantageous to plot data. It is also a better presentation mode, so the data in the table are plotted. This graph is shown in Figure 15.1.

It is seen that "it takes a little time for the process to get started," but thereafter, the uptake seems to be linear. It is not fruitful to dwell on why there is a lag time nor to speculate that it cannot be linear forever. The correct thing is to think simply at this stage and get the broad picture. One simply plots the part of the curve where there is moisture uptake. Why did the lag time happen? One can address that point later. The important point is that, in a certain range, there is a linear portion of the graph.

Even if the curves aren't quite linear, one should not be purist at this point, and some liberties may be taken. Sometimes a little "massaging" is not out of the question.

How does one get ideas? The slopes of the curves obviously increase with increasing relative humidity. Again, it is important to graph the

TABLE 15.1. Moisture Uptake Rates of a Drug Substance at Different Relative Humidities.

Time (Days)	50% Relative Humidity	61% Relative Humidity	84% Relative Humidity
0	0	0	0
1	0	0	0.62
2	0	0.38	1.15
3	0.25	0.9	1.9
4	0.41	1.25	2.35
5	0.55	1.55	
6	0.81		

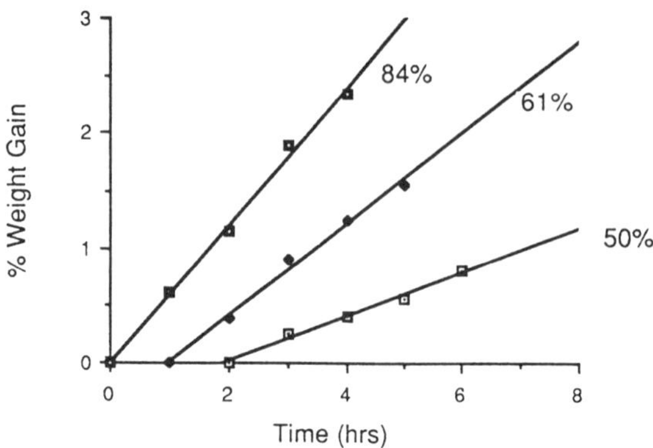

Figure 15.1 Data from Table 15.1.

trends one observes. So they are tabulated (Table 15.2), and the slopes are shown in a new graph (Figure 15.2).

The data do *not* lie on a good straight line, but again, one need not concern oneself too much with niceties at this point. The goal (a limited one at this point in time) is to find out at what relative humidity one can store the drug substance. Obviously, where the slope from Figure 15.1 would equal zero, the moisture uptake rate would equal zero, so if one could extrapolate the points to the x-axis, one could simply read off this "critical" relative humidity.

This is where the purist and thinker often trips him/herself up by saying that they couldn't possibly draw a line through the points. Of course, you can draw a line through the points. Not if you want to publish the data. What would you do then? Get more points, of course. But for the time being, why not draw a straight line? You don't have to show it to anyone. So Figure 15.3 shows this line, and it is, of course, not a panacea of precision.

It is, at best, a dubious plot. (The correlation coefficient is barely significant on the 90% level.) But it gives a very important piece of information. The RH-value that is being sought is probably between 30 and 40%.

So now one may rationally carry out a couple of more experiments, say about 35, 40, and 45, and when this is done, the data in Table 15.3 result. These are then entered onto a graph, and it is obvious that there is no moisture pickup at 35% RH. Do the other points lie on a straight line? One

TABLE 15.2. Slopes from Figure 15.1.

RH (%)	50	61	50
Slope (%/day)	0.19	0.40	0.60

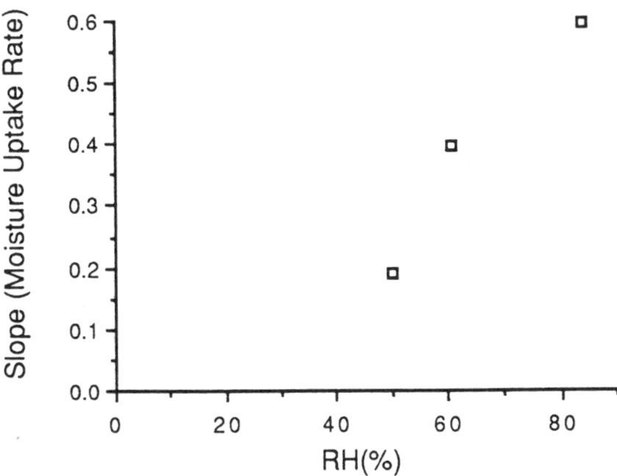

Figure 15.2 Slopes (moisture uptake rates) from Figure 15.1.

inconsistency would seem to be present in the data, in that the "high" point doesn't seem to lie on the line. But the scientist/formulator should say to him/herself that it doesn't matter; the linear points are quite linear, and they seem to say that the intersection is at 39% RH. So s/he will adopt a bit of leeway and say 35%. The data are there to show it.

As far as an industrial project, the question has been answered. The report is written and filed away. Great decisions are made based on it, in that the areas in which handling takes place must be below 35% RH. New buildings may have to be built. Dollars will be spent. Profits, hopefully, will rise.

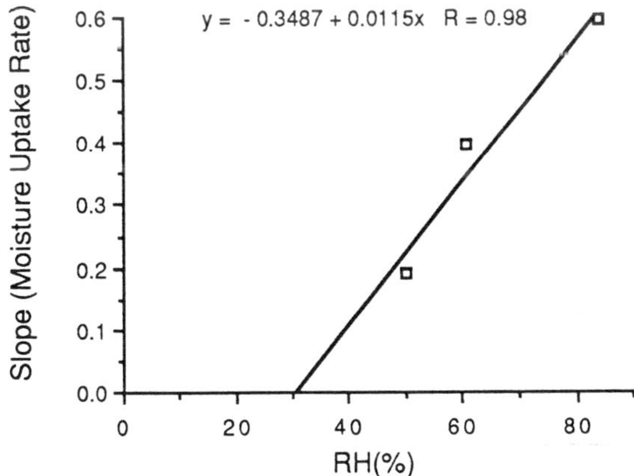

Figure 15.3 Figure 15.2 with line drawn.

TABLE 15.3. Slopes from Figure 15.1. The Italicized Numbers Have Been Added to the Experiments in Figure 15.1.

RH (%)	50	61	50	*35*	*40*	*45*
Slope (%/day)	0.19	0.40	0.60	*0*	*0.02*	*0.110*

15.6 THE SATURDAY AFTERNOON EXPERIMENT: THE QUICK-AND-DIRTY

The previous sections concentrate on a problem from the point of an industrial preformulation scientist. But what about an academic scientist. Would he do likewise?

In his case, he would ask himself the question, presumably through reading (maybe industrial consulting): What is hygroscopicity? He would want to design an experimental protocol, but before he did that, he would have to know a bit about his system. The way to orient oneself is to do a couple of experiments, e.g., the ones leading to Figure 15.1. This is what the late Professor Ed Garrett used to call a Saturday afternoon experiment, or a quick-and-dirty. Can you handle the system? Can you learn something from it? In an academic setting, you have the freedom of choice of materials, for instance, but this can be a deterrent. What if you had selected sand as your model compound? You would have learned that you ought to try something else.

So, in academe as well, the scientist/researcher would have arrived, finally, at Figure 15.4.

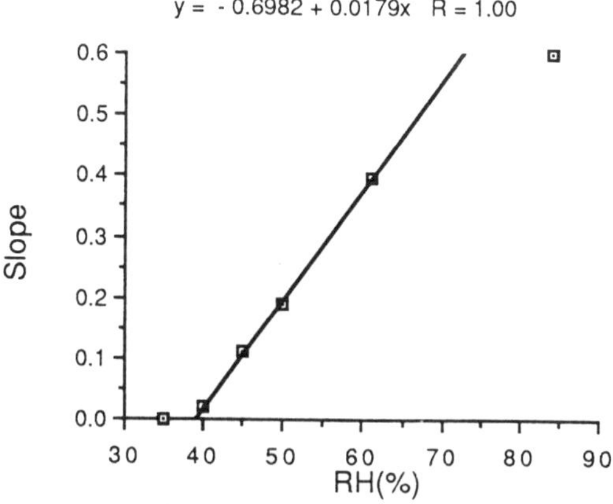

Figure 15.4 Figure 15.3 with more data added.

15.7 INITIAL CONCLUSIONS FROM THE GRAPH

The preformulation scientist or researcher will first of all set up an equation to describe Figure 15.4. The points on the graph are rates (moisture uptake rates), and they are linear in relative humidity beyond a certain point. So he writes

$$\text{Rate} = q(\text{RH} - \text{RH}_0) \tag{15.1}$$

That is a beginning. He refines this a bit by saying that, if M is the amount of water on 1 g of particles, then the rate is dM/dt, i.e.,

$$dM/dt = q(\text{RH} - \text{RH}_0) \tag{15.2}$$

Writing it that way may help or may not. We shall see.

15.8 THE INITIAL MODELING THOUGHTS: THE DOODLE

Once Figure 15.4 is arrived at, the scientist may want to repeat or add more points, but let us assume that the linearity of the plot prevails, and the question then is: What is really going on?

Why are the plots linear? Why do they "stop" at a certain relative humidity? To get a picture of what happens, it is best to draw or "doodle" one's visualization of the situation. In the following, the drawings and figures are, when they refer to such thoughts, drawn by hand on MacDraw and, hence, are not clean and perfect, and this is done on purpose. Often, such thoughts are done on a napkin in a restaurant or on toilet paper for that matter. How do ideas come? Only by steady thinking and reading, and at what point a possible path to the solution occurs is not predictable. But when a thought occurs, doodle it down.

In the case before us, we have particles and we have water vapor molecules, and somehow the water vapor molecules latch onto the surface in a predictable manner. So we doodle a particle and some water molecules and show them going on the surface (Figure 15.5).

The first question that arises is: Do the molecules adsorb onto the surface (like in an adsorption isotherm), or is there a layer of water on top of the particle?

So (and this thought may not occur immediately) the scientist looks for the consequences of its being a layer. If it were a layer of water, then the vapor pressure above it would be that of pure water, P_s, water's saturation pressure at the temperature of the experiment (T), or the relative humidity would be 100%. But if the relative humidity in the experiments is lower

TABLE 15.4. Moisture Uptake Rates at 65% of Four Mesh Cuts of the Drug Substance from Table 15.1 (Batch 1).

Mesh Cut Avg Particle Size (μm)	149	420	630	840
Moisture Uptake Rate (%/day)	0.6	0.25	0.125	0.1

It may take some time to figure it out, or it might be evident from the analogies found in mass transfer that the surface areas have to be comparable. So out s/he goes and measures the surface areas of the two samples that gave different slopes, and lo and behold, the rates are in the same ratio as the surface areas.

To be exacting, s/he now does the experiment with, for example, four mesh cuts of the drug substance, and he gets results as shown in Table 15.4.

And, again, the procedure to follow is to graph the data in their most native form, i.e., the uptake rate versus the particle diameter. This is done in Figure 15.6.

If the preformulator has *not* come to the conclusion that area is the important parameter, s/he might wonder how to transform a plot such as this. S/He would go through curve-fitting exercises, and surprise, surprise (!) plotting uptake rates versus the reciprocal of the particle diameter gives a straight plot (Figure 15.7). This shows the importance of curve-fitting skills!

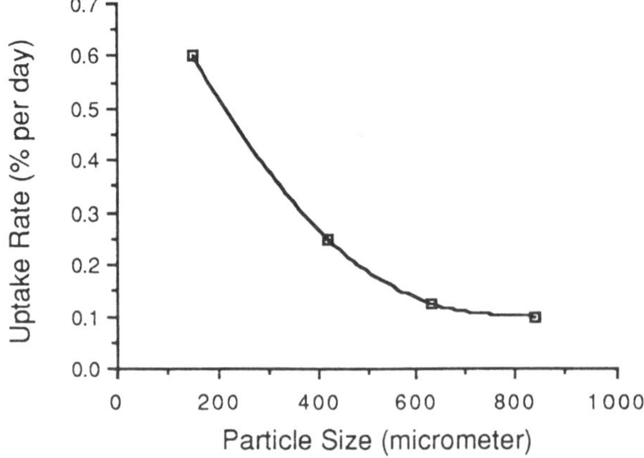

Figure 15.6 Data from Table 15.4.

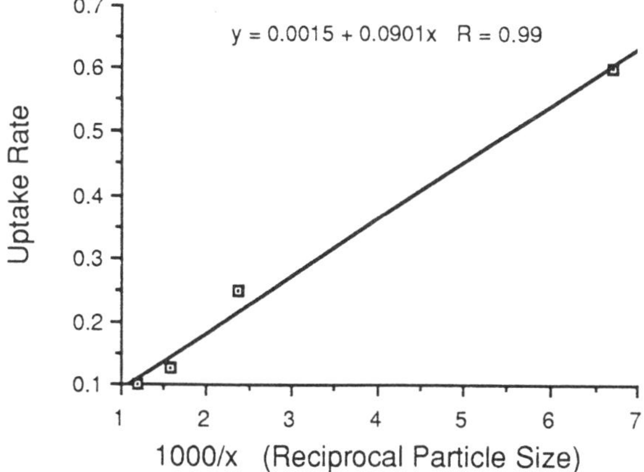

Figure 15.7 Uptake data from Table 15.4 plotted versus reciprocal diameter of the particle population.

Will s/he now in the report or publication simply record this fact as an amazing coincidence or what? If s/he has not come upon the area dependence, s/he might do the same experiment with another batch of the compound or with another substance, and s/he would find the same relationships.

The idea of the specific surface area being inversely proportional to the diameter may be a fact s/he knows, but even without knowing it, s/he may at this point suspect that it is, indeed, the surface area that is of importance, so the mesh cuts in Table 15.4 are subjected to surface area measurements with the results shown in Table 15.5.

The uptake rates are plotted versus specific surface area in Figure 15.8, and a reasonable linearity is obtained.

If one wants to add some "extras" to the writeup, one may plot the actual

TABLE 15.5. Moisture Uptake Rates at 65% of Four Mesh Cuts of the Drug Substance from Table 15.1 (Batch 1).

Mesh Cut				
Avg Particle Size (μm)	149	420	630	840
Moisture Uptake Rate (%/day)	0.6	0.25	0.125	0.1
Specific Surface Area (m^2/g)	3	1.3	1	0.5

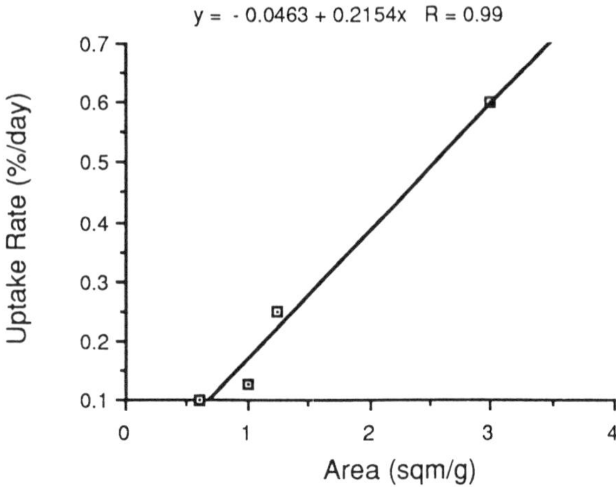

Figure 15.8 Data from Table 15.5.

surface areas versus $100/x$ (where x is diameter) and show linearity. This, again, is a side issue. But it should be tucked away for a "rainy day."

What if one did this for many substances? [The geometric surface area of a monodisperse particle size sample is (6/Density) × (weight in grams/diameter in cm).] Could one get information about particle *shape* in this way? This is noted because this is the way ideas come up. Dig for gold and you also find oil!

But back to the task at hand. The equation is now

$$dM/dt = q_2 A(P_{\text{atm}} - P_{\text{sat}}) \tag{15.4}$$

15.10 THE FINISHING TOUCHES

It should be decided that this is a good point to share one's up-to-date findings with the scientific community, and a publication (or internal report) should therefore be prepared.

This adds the concept of the area dependence to what has been said in the "publication" so far. Writing such as the following would be part of the article: "Having observed, as shown in Figure 1, the linearity of moisture uptake rates with time at different relative humidities and having demonstrated the validity of Equation (1), it seems clear that the moisture uptake rate would also be proportional to the surface area, A. To this end, samples of several compounds were exposed to a given relative humidity (65%) and the moisture uptake monitored. The moisture uptake rates are shown as a function of particle size, x, in Figure 2 [Figure 15.6], and this figure is indicative of the surface area dependence. The uptake rates were therefore plotted versus the actual surface areas of the different samples, and good linearity was observed as seen in Figure 3 [Figure 15.8]. . . ."

Now, having written it up, and again this is important, there is suddenly the realization that this has been done for one compound only. Also, some of the graphs could be refined by having more points. By looking at Figure 15.8, a point at a surface area of 2.5 m^2/g might make the graph a bit better.

The approach to take is *not* to repeat data with the substance already tested, but to (since one desires to do this for several substances) repeat the experiment with other suitable candidates.

Here one may draw from the experience gained with the first compound. Let us assume that the findings are the same. There may be a trend with solubility, but it is found to be inconsistent. Why? A little thought will guide the scientist back to his own equation, Equation (15.4). Both S and k might be different for different compounds. So the article ends with a statement such as: "Table 2 [not in this book] shows the effect of solubility on the transfer of moisture. If all the values of k were the same, then there should be a correlation with S. Since there is not, one might conclude that what is usually termed hygroscopicity contains both a kinetic (k) and a thermodynamic component (S)."

15.11 SCRUTINIZING THE SHORTCUTS TAKEN

It was stated previously that the point of the writing was a good resting point. Writing is always good because it shows where there are missing experiments, where there are illogical conclusions, where facets have been overlooked. So even during the process of modeling experience, it is advantageous to write, to write, and to write.

But as the experience has been progressing, thoughts occur—the serendipitous thoughts that may lead to other projects, as mentioned along the way, and also the simplifications that have been made in the model.

Coming back to Figure 15.1—and this is the basis for it all—there are aspects that have not been taken into account and points that have been assumed, tacitly assumed. Such assumptions should always be written down as they occur to the investigator. S/He may not have realized them at the onset, but they will occur as thoughts on the way. When they do, the tack is *not to start from square one, but to continue in the decided-on track,* and then to consider the additional thoughts when the first phase is finished.

A few assumptions made, but not stated, are listed in question form on the following page.

(1) Is the solution saturated, or is it a steady-state affair where as much drug dissolves as water is adsorbed, so that it is a steady-state concentration that occurs rather than saturation?
(2) Does heat of solution[22] give rise to a temperature that at the onset, is not constant?
(3) Is the relative humidity at the surface of the solid the same as in the surrounding atmosphere? There may be a pressure gradient from the atmosphere into the surface of the solid.

15.12 IT NEVER ENDS

Aside from these assumptions that would need clarification in further work, there is other work that presents itself as possible fields of investigation, for instance,

(1) The graphs, such as those in Figure 15.1, can be carried out for longer periods of time. They should eventually lead to solutions of the same vapor pressure as that of the atmosphere. This would be a good way of obtaining the aqueous vapor pressure versus concentration curve for a compound. It would be possible to see if it is "ideal" or not.
(2) The effect of temperature would be interesting. Here it should be able to tie in the data with the solubility-temperature curve of the compound.
(3) Verification of the assumption of saturation could be obtained through dissolution studies. If, indeed, it were a steady-state situation, then dissolution rate constants in stagnant fluid could be determined and may be compared with dissolution observed under the microscope.

And the list does not end there.

Modeling is like a breakthrough. Once a scientist has a hold on a system, one project leads to the next. And it never ends.

15.13 PROBLEMS

In the other chapters in the book where problems are included, they have been placed near the end of the chapter with answers following. Not so in this case, because to give problems in modeling and give the answer would defy the purpose.

First or all, there is not just one solution, and it is difficult, without

[22] This point has been investigated by VanCampen et al. (1980, 1983).

having the opportunity to do more experiments, to gauge the quality of one's model. The problems will, therefore, be presented as unanswered.

It is the hope of the author that this chapter will inspire scientists who have been hesitant, to go forward and do great things in modeling, and that the rest of the book has been of use to those who are already well versed in the field.

(1) Attempt to model the Heckel equation:

$$-\ln [\epsilon] = kP + q$$

where ϵ is the porosity of a compact made on a tablet machine at applied pressure p and where k and q are constants.

Develop a program that generates data according to the equation and show how these "experimental" data fit your model.

(2) A drug is an ester that hydrolyzes in solution:

$$RCOOR' + H_2O \rightarrow RCOOH + ROH$$

Write a program in BASIC describing the pH of an unbuffered solution as it decomposes. Or assume that the pH decreases linearly in time, and determine the decomposition profile of the compound as a function of time at a given temperature.

(3) The following data are obtained from a diametral hardness tester, where the failure strength is obtained by applying a force to the edge (wall) of the tablet. The thickness in Table 15.6 is the thickness of this "wall." Express the hardness as a logical parameter (e.g., stress).

(4) Assume that the ideal gas law is not known. Transform the variables in Table 15.7 in a logical way to establish the relationship between weight, pressure, volume, and temperature. Then use the parameter estimates as first estimates in nonlinear regression.

TABLE 15.6. Hardness Data.

Thickness, mm	Hardness (kP)
15	10.1
14.5	9.5
15.1	9.9
13.2	7.2
12.9	6.9
13.0	7.0
11.2	4.0
10.5	3.9
10.9	4.6

TABLE 15.7. Gas Properties.

Volume (liters)	Pressure (atm)	Temp (°C)	grams (of gas)
22.4	1	25	18
16.6	1.4	10	18
40.73	0.3	25	9
10	0.51	40	3.6
3	3.97	50	8.1
5	0.44	-5	1.8

15.14 REFERENCES

Carstensen, J. T. (1977), *Pharmaceutics of Solids and Solid Dosage Forms,* Wiley, NY, pp. 12–14.

Heckel, R. W., (1951), *Trans. Metal Soc. of AIME,* 221:671.

VanCampen, L., Zografi, G. and Carstensen, J. T., (1980), *Int. J. Pharm.,* 5:1.

VanCampen, L., Amidon, G. L., and Zografi, G., (1983), *J. Pharm. Sci.,* 72:1381, 1388, 1394.

CHAPTER 16

Concluding Remarks

The pharmaceutical sciences address two aspects of research: (a) problem solving and (b) elucidation of principles of (mostly) multi-component systems.

The way many researchers and consultants attack problems and projects is often based on folksy advice they have had in their pasts or, of course, of experiences they have had. Those of the author's can be summarized in interactions with colleagues of all ilks and are exemplified by the following events and principles:

(1) As a department head of the encapsulation department at Lederle Laboratories (then American Cyanamid Co.) in the 1950s, I was often confronted with telephone calls from others when advice on production problems was sought. My mentor then, John Vance, told me that you cannot discuss a problem rationally over the phone; you have to "go there and see for yourself," the lesson being that things get lost in translation. When one person says one thing, even a professionally similar listener may perceive the situation differently.

(2) Once, in a situation where a product would not handle well on filling equipment, I mentioned my frustration to my packaging colleague, Walter Rumpf, saying that I had had enough problems for one day. He responded, "God bless our problems; without them there would be no need for us."

(3) When I worked in Industry (1950–1967), I never lacked for problems. When I entered academe later in life, I had plenty of problems that had been unsolved for me in the past that I could tackle. But this is only true of someone who has been in Industry. If someone becomes a professor right out of school, he is liable to continue doing research in line with his own Ph.D. thesis for many years. As a colleague of mine once said, "We professors can solve any problem. Our dilemma is we don't know what the problems are."

(4) When one starts attacking a problem that one wants to solve, it is customary to do a literature search first. This is *almost* the correct approach. But such a search may leave one frustrated, feeling that everything that could possibly be done has already been done. In the words of the late and great Ed Garrett (U. Florida), it behooves one to do a "quick-and-dirty" or a "Saturday afternoon experiment," to get a feel for the system. "Everything" has never been done, and there is always room for more.

(5) A question often raised by students writing their required Grant Proposal (a requirement in many Ph.D. programs) is: "What do I write about? How do I get ideas?" I read a book in the 1950s called: *The Theory (or: Process?) of Mathematical Invention.* Later, I tried to locate it (having forgotten the author's name—he was Belgian), but I have never been able to find it. His observation was that he could think and think about the solution to a problem, not solve it, and then finally give up. Weeks or months later, at some unimportant moment in time (as he was stepping off a street car, for instance), the solution would come to him. So why did he do all the thinking in the first place? Because it is a necessary prerequisite. So thinking, thinking hard about a problem is a necessity.

(6) Finally, ideas come through reading and literature searching (after the "quick-and-dirty"). Here several pieces of advice are in order: Do not, at first, rely on computer searches. Go through twenty years of the three most pertinent journals in the field, either by index or page by page. A couple of weeks of work at this stage are a good investment.

Then do the computer search. For the academic researcher, the reason is one of serendipity because s/he often, in his/her reading, comes across other subject matter, which s/he should jot down, without going into detail. They may form the basis for the next project or may remind him/her of questions s/he has had in the past. In other words, they are idea #2, or indeed, s/he may abandon the first project entirely in favor of the second one.

We live in an age of protocols, and academically, there is no place for such an approach.

Industrially, it is different because the scientist cannot say, for instance, that "this compound is too difficult to assay; let me try another one." The compound in question is the one the company wants to market.

But here, also, a thorough search by hand is worthwhile, over and above a computer search, except that library searches in many companies are thought of as simply a way the scientist has of "goofing off." Not so!

(7) Finally, interaction with other scientists, actual collaboration, is a way to spawn ideas. The concept of "brainstorming" is an old one that is not used much today. Several people sequester themselves in a room for an unspecified time and throw out ideas for solving of a problem. The rules are:
- You can say anything without fear of someone saying, "That is stupid." Often, solutions come from the strangest approaches.
- The people in the group must trust one another. You cannot have someone in the group leave the meeting and take credit for something he thought of as a consequence of ideas having been spawned by other ideas.
- In other words, the group takes credit for whatever approach is successful, not the individual.

(8) And if all of the above fail, you can always steal someone else's idea. It happens.

APPENDICES

APPENDIX 1: AREAS UNDER THE NORMAL ERROR CURVE

TABLE A1. Areas under the Normal Error Curve.

Z	Area	Z	Area	Z	Area
-3.0	0.001	-1.0	0.159	1.0	0.841
-2.9	0.002	-0.9	0.184	1.1	0.864
-2.8	0.003	-0.8	0.212	1.2	0.885
-2.7	0.003	-0.7	0.242	1.3	0.903
-2.6	0.005	-0.6	0.274	1.4	0.919
-2.5	0.006	-0.5	0.309	1.5	0.933
-2.4	0.008	-0.4	0.345	1.6	0.945
-2.3	0.011	-0.3	0.382	1.7	0.955
-2.2	0.014	-0.2	0.421	1.8	0.964
-2.1	0.018	-0.1	0.460	1.9	0.971
-2.0	0.023	0.0	0.500	2.0	0.977
-1.9	0.029	0.1	0.540	2.1	0.982
-1.8	0.036	0.2	0.579	2.2	0.986
-1.7	0.045	0.3	0.618	2.3	0.989
-1.6	0.055	0.4	0.655	2.4	0.992
-1.5	0.067	0.5	0.691	2.5	0.994
-1.4	0.081	0.6	0.726	2.6	0.995
-1.3	0.097	0.7	0.758	2.7	0.997
-1.2	0.115	0.8	0.788	2.8	0.997
-1.1	0.136	0.9	0.816	2.9	0.998
				3.0	0.999

APPENDIX 2: Z-VALUES AS A FUNCTION OF AREA UNDER THE NORMAL ERROR CURVE

Appendix 2 shows the values of the area as a function of the Z-value. Frequently, the opposite is of value, and Appendix 2 shows the Z-value corresponding to a certain area.

TABLE A2. Z-Values as a Function of Area under the Normal Error Curve.

Area	Z	Area	Z	Area	Z
0	0	0.20	0.526	0.39	1.226
0.01	0.025	0.21	0.553	0.40	1.282
0.02	0.050	0.22	0.583	0.41	1.340
0.03	0.074	0.23	0.612	0.42	1.405
0.04	0.100	0.24	0.643	0.43	1.476
0.05	0.126	0.25	0.674	0.44	1.555
0.06	0.151	0.26	0.707	0.45	1.645
0.07	0.176	0.27	0.739	0.455	1.695
0.08	0.201	0.28	0.772	0.46	1.825
0.09	0.227	0.29	0.806	0.465	1.811
0.10	0.253	0.3	0.842	0.47	1.881
0.11	0.280	0.31	0.877	0.475	1.960
0.12	0.306	0.32	0.915	0.48	2.054
0.13	0.331	0.33	0.954	0.485	2.170
0.14	0.359	0.34	0.994	0.49	2.327
0.15	0.386	0.35	1.036	0.492	2.410
0.16	0.413	0.36	1.080	0.495	2.575
0.17	0.440	0.37	1.124	0.497	2.750
0.18	0.468	0.38	1.175	0.498	2.880
0.19	0.496			0.499	3.080

APPENDIX 3: TABLE OF STUDENT *t*-VALUES

TABLE A3. Student *t*-Values.

Degrees of Freedom	97.5% One Sided = 95% Two Sided	95% One Sided 90% Two Sided
1	12.706	6.3238
2	4.3027	2.9200
3	3.1825	2.3534
4	2.7764	2.1318
5	2.5706	2.0150
6	2.4469	1.9432
7	2.3646	1.8946
8	2.3060	1.8595
9	2.2622	1.8331
10	2.2281	1.8125
11	2.2010	1.7959
12	2.1788	1.7823
13	2.1604	1.7709
14	2.1448	1.7613
15	2.1315	1.7530
16	2.1199	1.7459
17	2.1098	1.7396
18	2.0019	1.7341
19	2.0930	1.7291
20	2.0860	1.7247
∞	1.96	1.645

APPENDIX 4: PROGRAMS FOR *t*-VALUES

TABLE A4a. Program for Calculating *t* (two-sided, 95% confidence or 90% one-sided).

```
885 INPUT "DF="; N2
888 IF N2 = 1 THEN T = 12.706
889 IF N2 = 2 THEN T = 4.303
890 IF N2 = 3 THEN T = 3.182
891 IF N2 = 4 THEN T = 2.776
892 IF N2 = 5 THEN T = 2.571
893 IF N2 = 6 THEN T = 2.447
894 IF N2 = 7 THEN T = 3.265
895 IF N2 >7 THEN T = 1.96 + (1/(-1.3489 +
(.42363*N2)))
910 PRINT N2, T
```

TABLE A4b. Output from Table A3. Student *t*-Values, 95% Two-Sided or 90% One-Sided.

df	df+2 *	t-value	t(approx)**
1	3		12.71
2	4		4.30
3	5		3.18
4	6		2.78
5	7	2.57	2.54
10	12	2.228	2.221
15	17	2.131	2.130
20	22	2.086	2.084
25	27	2.060	2.058
30	32	2.042	2.041
35	42	2.021	2.020
60	62	2000	2.000

*= N in least squares fitting of lines since df = N-2

**According to the Equation in Step 895

APPENDIX 5: *F*-VALUES ON THE 95% CONFIDENCE LEVEL

TABLE A5. *F*-Values on the 95% Confidence Level.

	Degrees of Freedom in the Numerator									
	1	2	3	4	5	6	7	8	9	10
d.f. in Denominator										
1	181	200	216	225	230	234	236	239	241	242
2	18.5	19.0	19.2	19.3	19.3	19.3	19.4	19.4	19.4	19.4
3	10.1	9.55	9.28	9.12	9.01	8.94	8.89	8.85	8.80	8.79
4	7.71	6.94	6.59	6.39	6.26	6.16	6.09	6.04	6.00	5.96
5	6.61	5.79	5.41	5.19	5.05	4.95	4.88	4.82	4.77	4.74
6	5.99	5.14	4.76	4.53	4.39	4.28	4.21	4.15	4.10	4.06
7	5.59	4.74	4.35	4.12	3.97	3.87	3.79	3.73	3.68	3.64
8	5.32	4.46	4.07	3.84	3.69	3.58	3.50	3.44	3.39	3.35
9	5.12	4.26	3.86	3.63	3.48	3.37	3.29	3.23	3.18	3.14
10	4.96	4.10	3.71	3.48	3.33	3.22	3.14	3.07	3.02	2.98

APPENDIX 6: *r*-STATISTIC FOR OUTLIERS

TABLE A6. *r*-Statistic for Outliers.

r-Type	No of Data	Upper Percentiles		
		0.90	0.95	0.98
		0.90	0.95	0.98
r	3	0.886	0.941	0.976
r_{10}	4	0.679	0.765	0.846
r_{10}	5	0.557	0.642	0.729
r_{10}	6	0.482	0.560	0.644
r_{10}	7	0.434	0.507	0.586
r_{11}	8	0.479	0.554	0.631
r_{11}	9	0.441	0.512	0.587
r_{11}	10	0.409	0.477	0.551
r_{21}	11	0.517	0.476	0.638
r_{21}	12	0.490	0.456	0.605
r_{21}	13	0.467	0.521	0.578
r_{22}	14	0.492	0.546	0.602
r_{22}	15	0.472	0.525	0.579

APPENDIX 7: STUDENTIZED RANGE, *q*

TABLE A7. Studentized Range, *q*, on the 95% Level.

t->	2	3	4	5	6	7	8	9	10
ν									
1	18	367	33	37	40	43	45	47	49
2	6.1	8.4	9.8	10.9	11.7	12.4	13.0	13.5	14
3	4.5	5.9	6.8	7.5	8.0	8.5	8.9	9.2	9.5
4	3.9	5.0	5.8	6.3	6.7	7.1	7.4	7.6	7.8
5	3.6	4.6	5.2	5.7	6.0	6.3	6.6	6.8	7.0
6	3.5	4.3	4.9	5.3	5.6	5.9	6.1	6.3	6.5
7	3.3	4.2	4.7	5.1	5.4	5.6	5.8	6.0	6.2
8	3.3	4.0	4.5	4.9	5.2	5.4	5.6	5.8	5.9
9	3.2	4.0	4.4	4.8	5.0	5.2	5.5	5.6	5.7
10	3.2	3.9	4.3	4.7	4.9	5.1	5.3	5.5	5.6

APPENDIX 8: CHI-SQUARED VALUES ON THE 2.5, 95, AND 97.5% CONFIDENCE LEVELS

TABLE A8. Chi-Squared Values on the 2.5, 95, and 97% Confidence Levels.

Degrees of Freedom	2.5%	95%	97.5%
1	0	4.852	5.024
2	0.506	5.991	7.378
3	0.216	7.815	9.348
4	0.484	9.488	11.143
5	0.831	11.07	12.832
6	1.237	12.592	14.449
7	1.690	14.067	16..013
8	2.180	15.507	17.535
9	2.700	16.919	19.023
10	3.247	18.307	20.481
11	3.186	19.675	21.920
12	4.404	21.026	32.336
13	5.009	22.362	24.736
14	5.629	23.685	26.119
15	6.262	24.996	27.488

APPENDIX 9: PROGRAM FOR GENERATING RANDOM NUMBERS IN BASIC

TABLE A9. Program for Generating Random Numbers in BASIC.

```
INPUT "NUMBER OF 16 DIGIT NUMBERS=";N
FOR Q = 1 TO N
PRINT (10*RND(1)) + 1
NEXT Q
```

Index